100 QUESTIONS IN CARDIOLOGY

100 QUESTIONS IN CARDIOLOGY

Edited by
Diana Holdright

Consultant Cardiologist, Department of Cardiology,
UCL Hospitals, London, UK

and

Hugh Montgomery
Honorary Consultant, UCL Hospitals Intensive Care Unit,
and
Lecturer in Cardiovascular Genetics, UCL Hospitals,
The Middlesex Hospital, London, UK

© BMJ Books 2001
BMJ Books is an imprint of the BMJ Publishing Group

First published in 2001
by BMJ Books, BMA House, Tavistock Square,
London WC1H 9JR

www.bmjbooks.com

British Library Cataloguing in Publication Data

A catalogue record for this book is available from the British Library

ISBN 0-7279-1489-8

Typeset by Saxon Graphics Ltd, Derby
Printed and bound by MPG Books Ltd, Bodmin, Cornwall.

Contents

Contents

Contents

Contributors

Prithwish Banerjee
Specialist Registrar in Cardiology, Hull and East Yorkshire Hospitals, Hull Royal Infirmary, Hull, UK

Matthew Barnard
Consultant Anaesthetist, UCL Hospitals, The Middlesex Hospital, London, UK

J Benhorin
Associate Chief, The Heiden Department of Cardiology, Bikur Cholim Hospital and The Hebrew University, Jerusalem, Israel

John Betteridge
Professor of Endocrinology and Metabolism, UCL Hospitals, The Middlesex Hospital, London, UK

Kieran Bhagat
Regional Facilitator (Cardiovascular Programme), World Health Organisation and Honorary Professor of Clinical Pharmacology, Medical School, University of Zimbabwe, Harare, Zimbabwe

Aidan Bolger
Clinical Research Fellow, Department of Cardiac Medicine, National Heart and Lung Institute, London, UK

David J Brull
British Heart Foundation Junior Fellow, UCL Cardiovascular Genetics, Rayne Institute, London, UK

R Cesnjevar
Cardiothoracic Surgeon, Great Ormond Street Hospital for Children NHS Trust, London, UK

Peter Clifton
Director Clinical Research Unit, CSIRO Health Sciences and Nutrition, Adelaide, Australia

John Cockcroft
General Practitioner, CAA Authorised Medical Examiner, Billericay Health Centre, Billericay, Essex, UK

Martin Cowie
Senior Lecturer in Cardiology and Honorary Consultant Cardiologist, University of Aberdeen and Grampian University Hospitals Trust, Department of Cardiology, Aberdeen Royal Infirmary, Aberdeen, UK

Seamus Cullen
Senior Lecturer, Department of Grown Up Congenital Cardiology, UCL Hospitals, The Middlesex Hospital, London, UK

Vincent S DeGeare
Lecturer, Great Ormond Street Hospital for Children NHS Trust, London, UK

Vic Froelicher
Consultant Cardiologist, Cardiology Division, Veterans Affairs Palo Alto Health Care System, Stanford University, California, USA

Anthony Gershlick
Professor of Medicine, Department of Academic Cardiology, University of Leicester, UK

Cindy L Grines
Director of the Cardiac Catheterization Laboratories, Division of Cardiology, William Beaumont Hospital, Royal Oak, Michigan, USA

Suzanna Hardman
Senior Lecturer in Cardiology with an interest in Community Cardiology, University College London Medical School, and Honorary Consultant Cardiologist, the UCL and Whittington Hospitals
Address for correspondence: UCLMS (Whittington campus), Academic & Clinical Department of Cardiovascular Medicine, Whittington Hospital, London, UK

Martin Paul Hayward
Cardiothoracic Surgeon, The Austin and Repatriation Medical Centre, Melbourne, Australia

Daniel E Hillman
Professor and Chair, Department of Pharmacy Practice, Creighton University, Omaha, Nebraska, USA

Aroon Hingorani
Senior Lecturer in Clinical Pharmacology and Therapeutics, British Heart Foundation Intermediate Fellow, Centre for Clinical Pharmacology, UCL, Rayne Institute, London, UK

Diana Holdright
Consultant Cardiologist, Department of Cardiology, UCL Hospitals, The Middlesex Hospital, London, UK

Rachael James
Cardiology SpR, The Royal Sussex County Hospital Brighton, Brighton, UK

Roy M John
Associate Director, Cardiac Electrophysiology Laboratory, Lahey Clinic Medical Center, Burlington, MA, USA

Robin Kanagasabay
SpR Cardiothoracic Surgery, St George's Hospital Medical School, London, UK

RA Kenny
Head of Department of Medicine (Geriatric), University of Newcastle Upon Tyne, Institute for Health of the Elderly, Royal Victoria Infirmary, Newcastle Upon Tyne, UK

Brendan Madden
Consultant Cardiothoracic and Transplant Surgeon, Cardiothoracic Transplant Unit, St George's Hospital, London, UK

Kenneth W Mahaffey
Assistant Professor of Medicine, Duke Clinical Research Institute, Durham, NC, USA

Niall G Mahon
Specialist Registrar in Cardiology, St George's Hospital Medical School, London, UK

Joseph F Malouf
Associate Professor, Mayo Medical School, and Consultant, Division of Cardiovascular Diseases and Internal Medicine, Mayo Clinic, Rochester, Minnesota, USA

Richard Mansfield
Lecturer in Cardiology, Cardiovascular Repair and Remodeling Group, Middlesex Hospital, London, UK

W McKenna
Registrar in Cardiology, St George's Hospital Medical School, London, UK

Hugh Montgomery
Honorary Consultant, UCL Hospitals Intensive Care Unit, and Lecturer in Cardiovascular Genetics, UCL Hospitals, London, UK

Marc R Moon
Assistant Professor of Cardiothoracic Society Department of
Cardiothoracic Surgery, Washington University School of
Medicine, St Louis, Missouri, USA

Stan Newman
Professor of Psychology, Deptartment of Psychological Medicine,
UCL Hospitals, The Middlesex Hospital, London, UK

Petros Nihoyannopoulos
Senior Lecturer and Consultant Cardiologist, Cardiology
Department, Imperial College School of Medicine, National Heart
and Lung Institute, Hammersmith Hospital, London, UK

Michael S Norrell
Consultant Cardiologist, Hull and East Yorkshire Hospitals, Hull
Royal Infirmary, Hull, UK

Lionel H Opie
Co-Director, Cape Heart Centre and Medical Research Council,
Inter-University Cape Heart Group, University of Cape Town,
and Consultant Physician, Groote Schuur Hospital, Cape Town,
South Africa

Diarmuid O'Shea
Consultant Physician, Department of Geriatric Medicine, St
Vincent's University Hospital, Dublin, Ireland

Krishna Prasad
Specialist Registrar in Cardiology, Department of Cardiology,
University of Wales College of Medicine, Cardiff, UK

Liz Prvulovich
Consultant Physician in Nuclear Medicine, Institute of Nuclear
Medicine, Middlesex Hospital, London, UK

Henry Purcell
Senior Fellow in Cardiology, Royal Brompton and Harefield NHS
Trust, London, UK

Michael Schachter
Senior Lecturer in Clinical Pharmacology, Department of Clinical
Pharmacology, Imperial College School of Medicine, and
Honorary Consultant Physician, St Mary's Hospital, London, UK

Rakesh Sharma
Clinical Research Fellow, Department of Cardiac Medicine,
National Heart and Lung Institute, London, UK

Alistair Slade
Consultant Cardiologist, Royal Cornwall Hospitals Trust, Treliske Hospital, Truro, Cornwall, UK

Simon Sporton
Specialist Registrar in Cardiology, Department of Cardiology, St Bartholomew's Hospital, London, UK

Mark Squirrell
Senior Technician, Department of Cardiology, UCL Hospitals, The Middlesex Hospital, London, UK

Matthew Streetly
Specialist Registrar in Haematology, Department of Haematology, University College Hospital, London, UK

Jan Stygall
Clinical Psychologist, The Middlesex Hospital, London, UK

DP Taggart
Consultant Cardiothoracic Surgeon, John Radcliffe Hospital, Oxford, UK

Sara Thorne
Consultant Cardiologist, Department of Cardiology, Queen Elizabeth Hospital, Birmingham

Adam D Timmis
Consultant Cardiologist, Department of Cardiology, London Chest Hospital, London, UK

Tom Treasure
Consultant Cardiothoracic Surgeon, Department of Cardiothoracic Surgery, St George's Hospital, London, UK

Victor T Tsang
Consultant Cardiothoracic Surgeon, Great Ormond Street Hospital for Children NHS Trust, London, UK

Jonathan Unsworth-White
Consultant Cardiothoracic Surgeon, Department of Cardiothoracic Surgery, Derriford Hospital, Plymouth, Devon, UK

Peter Wilson
Consultant Microbiologist, Department of Clinical Microbiology, University College Hospital, London, UK

Introduction

This book differs from most other available cardiology texts. We have designed it to provide didactic answers to specific questions, wherever possible. Some are everyday questions. Others deal with less common situations, where an answer is often not readily found. The book is suitable for all grades of doctor, cardiologist and physician alike.

Responses have been kept as brief as possible and practical. A few important topics defied our editorial culling and were given more space. The aim was not to review the entire literature, but rather to present the conclusions which that author has reached from such evaluation, combined with experience. Where helpful or necessary, a few relevant references have been provided with the answer.

We hope that the text can be read in several ways to suit the reader – in one go, referred to on the wards or in clinic or dipped into for pleasure and education. The short question and answer format should permit such an approach.

We have tried to produce a selection of topics spanning most aspects of cardiovascular disease but there will, of course, be "obvious" questions which we have not posed. Please write to us c/o BMJ Books, BMA House, Tavistock Square, London WC1H 9JR, with any suggestions for questions you would like to see answered in a future edition. Finally, because the answers given are "personal" to each author, you may disagree with some responses. Please feel free to do so. This is not a set of guidelines set in stone.

Diana Holdright and Hugh Montgomery

Acknowledgement
We would like to acknowledge Dr Chris Newman whose initial suggestion led to this book.

1 What are the cardiovascular risks of hypertension?

Aroon Hingorani

The risk of death, stroke and coronary heart disease (CHD) increases continuously with increasing BP with no evidence of a threshold. The excess risk of stroke and CHD associated with BP differences of varying degrees is illustrated in Table 1.1.

Table 1.1   Effect of a sustained difference in BP on risk of stroke and CHD

Difference in usual		% increase in risk of	
SBP (mmHg)	DBP (mmHg)	Stroke	CHD
9	5	34	21
14	7.5	46	29
19	10	56	37

Meta-analysis of outcome trials shows that the reduction in risk achieved by antihypertensive treatment is approximately constant whatever the starting BP. Antihypertensive treatment producing a 5–6mmHg fall in DBP results in an approximately 36% reduction in stroke and a 16% reduction in CHD. Greater BP lowering would be expected to achieve greater risk reductions. Although the observed reduction in stroke risk from intervention trials is commensurate with that predicted by observational studies, the observed reduction in CHD risk is less than that expected (see Table 1.2). The reason for this discrepancy is unclear but might reflect: a clustering of additional cardiovascular risk factors (for example diabetes and hypercholesterolaemia) in hypertensive subjects; an adverse effect of some antihypertensive drugs (e.g. thiazides and β blockers) on plasma lipids; or the effect of pre-existing end-organ damage.

Table 1.2   Reductions in stroke and CHD risk resulting from a 5–6 mmHg reduction in BP

	Reduction in risk (%)	
	Expected	Observed
Stroke	35–40	31–45
CHD	20–25	8–23

Further reading

McMahon S. Blood pressure and risks of cardiovascular disease. In: Swales JD, ed. *Textbook of hypertension.* Oxford: Blackwell Scientific,1994:46.

Collins R, Peto R. Antihypertensive drug therapy. Effects on stroke and coronary heart disease. In: Swales JD, ed. *Textbook of hypertension.* Oxford: Blackwell Scientific, 1994:1156.

2 Is 24 hour blood pressure monitoring necessary, and what do I do with the information?

Kieran Bhagat

Patients with evidence of target organ damage, previous cardio-vascular events, high outpatient blood pressure, and older age are at high risk of developing vascular complications of hypertension. They are therefore likely to require antihypertensive treatment, irrespective of the 24 hour blood pressure profile. Ambulatory monitoring is therefore generally reserved for the assessment of those patients with mild hypertension without evidence of cardiovascular damage (possible "white coat" hypertension), hypertension that appears to be drug-resistant and in the assessment of antihypertensive treatment, particularly with symptoms suggestive of hypotension.

What do I do with the information from a 24 hour ambulatory BP result?

One problem associated with the use of ambulatory blood pressure monitoring in clinical practice has been the lack of internationally accepted reference values. Population studies have been used to define normal ambulatory blood pressure ranges, according to age and sex, and it is now possible to plot 24 hour blood pressures for each patient and determine if they fall within these accepted bands. The disadvantage of this method has been that many of the earlier published data were not obtained from population-based samples. Nonetheless, there are more than 30 cross-sectional studies that have linked ambulatory blood pressure to target organ damage using the parameters of left ventricular hypertrophy, microalbuminuria, retinal hypertensive changes and cerebrovascular disease. These studies have revealed ambulatory blood pressure to be a more sensitive predictor of target organ damage than single casual measurements, and it has been assumed that these surrogate end points of target organ involvement can be extrapolated to the ultimate end points of cardiac or cerebrovascular death and morbidity.

"White coat" hypertensives

The clinical significance of white coat hypertension has yet to be established. Some echocardiographic studies of left ventricular size have reported that people with white coat hypertension have similar indices to normotensive people, and one follow up study has even suggested that they have a similar prognosis. In contrast, some studies have reported that left ventricular dimensions in white coat hypertension are somewhere between those of normotension and sustained hypertension.

Dippers and non-dippers

The significance of average night time blood pressure readings remains equally uncertain. Stroke, silent cerebrovascular disease, and left ventricular hypertrophy are more common in patients who do not demonstrate the normal nocturnal fall in blood pressure, and this has led to the assumption that non-dipper status is an independent predictor of cardiovascular morbidity and mortality. There are a number of potential problems that may complicate this interpretation. Vascular disease itself could impair nocturnal blood pressure fall through impairment of cardiovascular reflexes. It remains uncertain whether this non-dipper status genuinely reflects a greater daily blood pressure load or whether it merely means that the patient did not sleep as soundly, having been disturbed by the inflation of the blood pressure cuff.

The results of a number of large scale studies of ambulatory blood pressure and prognosis are awaited. These include the European study OVA, the study on ambulatory blood pressure and treatment of hypertension (APTH), the SAMPLE study and the ABP arm of the European Working Party on High Blood Pressure Syst-Eur study.

Further reading

Clement D, De Buyzere M, Duprez D. Prognostic value of ambulatory blood pressure monitoring. *J Hypertens* 1994;**12**: 857–64.

Davies RJO, Jenkins NE, Stradling JR. Effects of measuring ambulatory blood pressure on sleep and on blood pressure during sleep. *BMJ* 1994;**308**: 820–3.

Devereux RB, Pickering TG. Relationship between the level, pattern and variability of ambulatory blood pressure and target organ damage in hypertension. *J Hypertens* 1991;**9**(suppl 8): S34–8.

3 Who should be screened for a cause of secondary hypertension? How do I screen?

Kieran Bhagat

The clinical context and the outcome of investigations that should be carried out on all hypertensive patients will determine who should be investigated for secondary causes of hypertension.

Routine tests that should be performed

- *Urinalysis*. Proteinuria is suggestive of underlying renal damage or a causative lesion within the kidney.
- *Routine biochemistry*. This may suggest the presence of renal dysfunction (urea, creatinine, uric acid) or underlying endocrine disease (Conn's, Cushing's, hyperparathyroidism).
- *Electrocardiography*. This may show the effects of long standing or poorly controlled hypertension (left ventricular hypertrophy, left axis deviation).

Further testing

If routine testing reveals abnormalities or the patient has been referred for "resistant hypertension" then further investigations are justified. These should be determined by clinical suspicion (for example, symptoms or signs of phaeochromocytoma, Cushingoid appearance etc.) and the outcome of routine investigations (for example proteinuria, haematuria, hypokalaemia etc.).

- *Urinalysis*. 24 hour quantification of protein, electrolytes, and creatinine clearance.
- *Radiological*. Initially, ultrasound examination of the abdomen screens renal size, anatomy and pelvicalyceal disease. Computerised tomography of the abdomen scan has greater sensitivity for adrenal tumours and phaeochromocytomas. MIBG scanning will help identify extra-adrenal phaeochromocytoma. Renal angiography will identify renal artery stenosis.
- *Renal biopsy* should be performed if microscopy or plasma immunological screening is suggestive of systemic inflammatory or renovascular disease.

- *Endocrine investigations.* 24 hour urinary cortisol (Cushing's syndrome), 24 hour noradrenaline/adrenaline/dopamine (catecholamine-secreting tumours), and plasma renin and aldosterone (Conn's syndrome) may all be warranted.

4 What blood pressure should I treat, and what should I aim for when treating a 45 year old, a 60 year old, a 75 year old or an 85 year old?

Aroon Hingorani

Who to treat

The primary aim of blood pressure (BP) treatment is to reduce the risk of stroke and CHD. Assuming secondary causes of hypertension have been excluded, the decision to treat a particular level of BP is based on an assessment of the risk of stroke, coronary heart disease (CHD) and hypertensive renal disease in the individual patient.

All patients with evidence of target organ damage (left ventricular hypertrophy, retinopathy, or hypertensive nephropathy) are considered to be at high risk and should receive treatment whatever the level of BP. Similarly, all patients who have previously suffered a stroke or CHD should have their BP lowered if it is above 140/90mmHg.

Difficulties arise in those without end-organ damage or a previous cardiovascular event. Guidelines in the UK have advocated antihypertensive treatment for sustained BP levels above 160/100mmHg since in these individuals the risks of stroke and renal disease are unacceptably high. Absolute risk of stroke or CHD depends, however, not only on BP but also on the combination of other risk factors (age, gender, total cholesterol, HDL-cholesterol, smoking, diabetes, and left ventricular hypertrophy). Their synergistic interaction in any individual makes universal application of BP thresholds perhaps inappropriate and some individuals with BP >140/90mmHg will benefit from treatment. Recent guidelines on treatment have also advocated a global assessment of risk rather than focusing on individual risk factors. The risk of stroke or CHD in an individual can be calculated using tables[1] or computer programmes[2] based on a validated risk function (for example Framingham Risk Equation). Having calculated absolute risk (based on the variables above), one has to decide what level of risk is worth treating. A low threshold for treatment will result in a larger number of individuals exposed to antihypertensive drugs and a higher cost, but a greater number of cardiovascular events saved. Meta-analysis has shown that (for a given level of BP lowering) the relative reduction in stroke and CHD is constant whatever the starting level of BP. Thus, the absolute benefit from BP lowering depends on the initial level of risk. A threshold *cardiovascular event* risk of 2% per year has been advocated by some[1] and equates to treating 40 individuals for five years to save one cardiovascular event (myocardial infarction, stroke, angina or cardiovascular death).

Young patients

Since age is a major determinant of absolute risk, treatment thresholds based on absolute risk levels will tend to postpone treatment to older ages. However, younger patients with elevated BP who have a low absolute risk of stroke and CHD exhibit greatly elevated *relative risks* of these events compared to their normotensive age-matched peers. Deciding on the optimal age of treatment in such individuals presents some difficulty and the correct strategy has yet to be determined.

Elderly patients

The absolute risk of CHD and stroke in elderly hypertensive patients is high and, consequently, the absolute benefit from treatment is much greater than in younger patients. Decisions to treat based on absolute risk are therefore usually straightforward. However, there is little in the way of firm trial evidence for the benefits of treatment in individuals aged more than 80. In these patients, decisions could be made on a case-by-case basis taking into account biological age.

What to aim for

Although it might be assumed that the lower the BP the lower the risk of stroke and CHD, some studies have described a J-shaped relationship between BP and cardiovascular events, where the risk of an adverse outcome rises slightly at the lower end of the BP range. However, in the large Hypertension Optimal Treatment (HOT) study[3] lowering BP to 130–140/80–85 mmHg was safe. While there was no additional advantage of lowering BP below these levels (except possibly in diabetic subjects), there was also no evidence of a J-shaped phenomenon in this large trial.

References
1 New Zealand guidelines and tables available at http: //www.nzgg.org.nz
2 Hingorani AD, Vallance P. A simple computer programme for guiding management of cardiovascular risk factors and prescribing. *BMJ* 1999;**318**: 101–5
3 Hansson L, Zanchetti A, Carruthers SG *et al*. Effects of intensive blood pressure lowering and low-dose aspirin in patients with hypertension: principal results of the HOT trial. *Lancet* 1998;**351**: 1755–62.

Further reading
Ramsay LE et al. British Hypertension Society guidelines for hypertension management 1999: summary. *BMJ* 1999;**319**: 630–5.

5 Is one treatment for hypertension proven to be better than another in terms of survival?

Kieran Bhagat

In terms of efficacy, there is no evidence that any one class of anti-hypertensive is superior to another at standard doses used as monotherapy. All agents reduce blood pressure by a similar amount (approximately 5–10mmHg). However, if one assesses the large outcome trials (in terms of survival) then only the diuretics are well supported in showing reduction in mortality. The beta blockers have **not** been shown to reduce mortality. The oft-quoted MRC trial in elderly people used atenolol and did not reduce mortality when compared to placebo.[1] Indeed, cardio-vascular mortality seemed to increase in the atenolol group. In the Swedish trial in elderly patients with hypertension,[2] in which mortality was reduced, initial beta blockade was one of the arms of treatment, but over two thirds of patients received an added diuretic. (If the proposal is that combined treatment with beta blockade and diuretic can reduce mortality then there are indirect supporting data from the Swedish trial.) In the MRC trial in middle-aged people, propranolol had only modest effects in non-smokers and conferred little or no benefit in smokers. Mortality was not decreased, and the trial was not powered for mortality. Nonetheless it can be convincingly argued that end points such as reduction in stroke are important and that the beta blockers have been shown to reduce the incidence of neurovascular events in several trials. By contrast there is already one good outcome study with a calcium blocker[3] but no outcome studies in essential hypertension in the elderly with ACE inhibitors, nor are there any in younger age groups. In spite of the above there still remain compelling reasons to prescribe a certain class of antihypertensive agent in patients that may have additional problems. For example, one might prescribe an ACE inhibitor to those with type 1 diabetes with proteinuria, or those with hypertension and heart failure. Similarly it might be equally cogent to prescribe a calcium antagonist in systolic hypertension in the elderly.

References
1 MRC Working Party. Medical Research Council trial of treatment of hypertension in older adults: principal results. *BMJ* 1992;**304**: 405–12.

2 Dahlof B, Lindholm LH, Hansson L *et al.* Morbidity and mortality in the Swedish trial in old patients with hypertension (STOP-hypertension). *Lancet* 1991;**338**: 1281–5.

3 Staessen JA, Fagard R, Thijs L *et al.* Randomised double-blind comparison of placebo and active treatment for older patients with isolated systolic hypertension (Syst-Eur Trial). *Lancet* 1997; **350**: 754–64.

6 It was once suggested that calcium channel blockers might be dangerous for treating hypertension. Is this still true?

Kieran Bhagat

Innumerable editorials, reviews and letters have been written on the calcium channel blocker controversy that started with the publication of the case-control study by Psaty *et al* in 1995[1] and the subsequent meta-analysis of Furberg *et al* in the same year.[2] They reported a greater increase in the risk of myocardial infarction among those taking short-acting calcium channel blockers than amongst those taking diuretics or beta-blockers. The risk was greatest at higher doses of nifedipine. Other concerns relate to an increase in gastrointestinal haemorrhage, bleeding in relation to surgery and cancer. Since then three further case-control studies have not found an association between calcium channel blockers and adverse cardiovascular outcome, while a leash of prospective trials have added greatly to the quality of the data available on this issue.

There is general consensus that short-acting dihydropyridines should not be given to patients with ischaemic heart disease. The position in hypertension is less clear. There do seem to be grounds for concern about short acting dihydropyridines relative to other treatments. The recent case-control studies do not seem to raise the same concerns with long-acting agents, at least from the point of view of adverse cardiovascular outcomes. However, the real safety profile of these agents in hypertension will not be known until many ongoing prospective randomised trials such as ALLHAT report.[3] Despite the absence of these trials a prudent interim approach would be to restrict the use of calcium antagonists to the newer slow-release formulations that, by virtue of their ability to attain more gradual and sustained plasma levels, do not evoke a reactive sympathetic activation.

References
1 Psaty BM, Heckbert SR, Koepsell TD *et al*. The risk of myocardial infarction associated with antihypertensive drug therapies. *JAMA* 1995; **274**: 620–5.
2 Furberg CD, Psaty BM, Meyer JV. Nifedipine. Dose-related increase in mortality in patients with coronary heart disease.*Circulation* 1995; **92**: 1326–31.

3 Cavis BR, Cutler JA, Gordon DJ *et al*. Rationale and design for the anti-hypertensive and lipid lowering treatment to prevent heart attack trial (ALLHAT). *Am J Hypertens* 1996; **9**: 342–60.

7 How can I outline a management plan for the patient with essential hypertension?

Aroon Hingorani

A management plan for the initial assessment, investigation and follow up of a patient presenting with elevated blood pressure is presented below.

INITIAL ASSESSMENT
- **Measure BP***
- **History (including drug and family history) and examination**
- **Baseline screen for secondary causes of hypertension****:
  urinalysis, creatinine and electrolytes
- **Assessment of end-organ damage*****:
  ECG, fundoscopy
- **Assessment of other cardiovascular risk factors:**
  age, gender, BP, total and HDL-cholesterol
  ECG-LVH, diabetes, smoking status

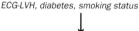

INSTITUTE LIFESTYLE MODIFICATIONS
- **Salt** (sodium restriction from 10g/d to 5g/d expect 5/3 mmHg reduction in BP)
- **Alcohol** (change depends on amount consumed)
- **Weight** (expect 1-2 mmHg BP reduction for every kg lost)
- **Aerobic exercise** (4/3 mmHg reduction for thrice weekly aerobic exercise)
- **Smoking cessation** (consider nicotine replacement)

COMPUTE CARDIOVASCULAR RISK
Use BP level and estimates of absolute and****
relative cardiovascular disease risk**** to guide:
- **Anti-hypertensive drug therapy**
  initial treatment with thiazide diuretic or beta blocker unless contraindicated or not tolerated
- **Cholesterol lowering with statins**
  consider aspirin

REVIEW
- Adequacy of treatment: BP and cholesterol target
- Side effects from treatment
- Lifestyle modifications

*   Sitting position. Mean of 2-3 measurements over 4–6 weeks unless severity of BP dictates earlier treatment.
**   Abnormalities identified from history, examination or baseline screen dictate further investigation to confirm/exclude renal parenchymal, renovascular, endocrine or other secondary causes of hypertension.
***   The presence of hypertensive retinopathy or LVH is an indication for BP lowering irrespective of the absolute BP level.
****For references to risk calculators see Qu4, page 7.

Reference: Vallance P. CME Cardiology II. Hypertension, *J Roy Coll Phys Lon* 1999; **33**: 119-23

8 How do I manage the patient with malignant hypertension?

Aroon Hingorani

Malignant hypertension was originally defined as hypertension in association with grade IV retinopathy (papilloedema), although it is now clear that hypertension associated with grade III retinopathy (retinal haemorrhages without papilloedema) shares the same poor prognosis. The identification of malignant hypertension should prompt an urgent and active search for secondary causes of hypertension, particularly renal disease (acute renal failure must be excluded), renovascular disease and phaeochromocytoma.

Management is based on the published experience from case series rather than randomised controlled trials. In the absence of hypertensive heart failure, aortic dissection or fits and confusion (hypertensive encephalopathy), bed rest and oral antihypertensive treatment are the mainstays of management, the aim being to reduce the diastolic blood pressure gradually to 100mmHg in the first few hours of presentation. Too rapid reduction in BP may precipitate "watershed" cerebral infarction. Oral therapy with β-adrenoceptor blockers (e.g. atenolol 50–100mg) ± a thiazide diuretic (e.g. bendrofluazide 2.5mg) will lower the blood pressure smoothly in most patients. There is less experience with newer antihypertensive agents. Nifedipine given via the sublingual route may produce a rapid and unpredictable reduction in BP and should be avoided. Similarly, angiotensin-converting enzyme inhibitors should also be avoided because of the risk of first dose hypotension. Older drugs such as hydralazine (25–50mg 8 hourly), or methyldopa (10–20mg 8 hourly) have been used successfully and are an alternative in individuals in whom β-adrenoceptor blockers are contraindicated.

Hypertensive encephalopathy (headache, fits, confusion, nausea and vomiting) demands intensive care, intra-arterial BP monitoring and a more urgent, but nevertheless controlled, blood pressure reduction with parenteral antihypertensive therapy. Labetalol (initial dose 15mg/hr) or sodium nitroprusside (initial dose 10 micrograms/min) are effective and readily titratable agents. The aim is to titrate the dose upwards to produce a controlled reduction in diastolic blood pressure to 100mmHg over 1–2 hours. For hypertensive encephalopathy in the context of pre-eclampsia, intravenous magnesium sulphate is a specific therapy. The presence of focal neurological signs should prompt a CT head scan to exclude haemorrhagic stroke or subarachnoid haemorrhage, in which case nimodipine should be started.

9 Which asymptomatic hypercholesterolaemic patients benefit from lipid-lowering therapy? What cholesterol level should I aim for?

John Betteridge

Recently two major primary prevention trials with statins, WOSCOPS[1] in hypercholesterolaemic men and AFCAPS/TEX-CAPS[2] in healthy men and women with average cholesterol and below average HDL cholesterol, have demonstrated highly significant reductions in CHD events. Although benefit extends to those at low absolute risk of an event it is sensible to reserve pharmacological therapy for those at highest risk. Recent joint recommendations of the British Cardiac Society, British Hyperlipidaemia Association and British Hypertension Society[3] suggest treatment (as a minimum) for an absolute risk of 30% or greater over 10 years with the ultimate objective of treating those with risk exceeding 15%. Goals of therapy are total cholesterol less than 5.0mmol/l (LDL-cholesterol <3.0mmol/l). Risk charts based on the Framingham prospective population data taking into account blood pressure, age, smoking status, diabetes and total cholesterol to HDL ratio are provided. These charts do not apply to individuals with severe hypertension, familial dyslipidaemia or diabetic patients with associated target organ damage who should receive statin therapy.

References

1 Shepherd J, Cobbe SM, Ford I *et al.* for the West of Scotland Coronary Prevention Study Group. Prevention of coronary heart disease with pravastatin in men with hypercholesterolaemia. *N Engl J Med* 1995; **333**: 1301–7.

2 Downs GR, Clearfield M, Weiss S *et al.* Primary prevention of acute coronary events with lovastatin in men and women with average cholesterol levels: results of AFCAPS/TEXCAPS. Air Force/Texas coronary atherosclerosis study. *JAMA* 1998; **279**: 1615–22.

3 Joint British recommendations on prevention of coronary heart disease in clinical practice. British Cardiac Society, British Hyperlipidaemia Association, British Hypertension Society endorsed by the British Diabetic Association. *Heart* 1998; **80 (suppl 2)**: S1–S29.

10 Which patients with coronary disease have been proven to benefit from pharmacological intervention? What lipid levels should I aim for?

John Betteridge

Three major statin trials (4S[1], CARE[2] and LIPID[3]) involving approximately 18,000 patients have provided unequivocal evidence of benefit of cholesterol-lowering in patients with established coronary heart disease (CHD, angina, unstable angina, post-myocardial infarction). The question might be better phrased, which CHD patient should not receive statins, as the overwhelming majority are likely to show substantial benefit. Debate remains concerning the optimal treatment goal for LDL and the level at which treatment should be initiated. The lesson from interpopulation epidemiology is that there is no threshold effect for cholesterol and CHD and the relationship is maintained at low levels. Furthermore, in LIPID the cholesterol inclusion criteria went down to 4mmol/l. The recent joint British guidelines suggest that treatment should be initiated at a total cholesterol >5mmol/l (LDL >3mmol/l) and the goal should be cholesterol <5 and LDL <3mmol/l. In the American Heart Association guidelines the goal of therapy is an LDL cholesterol <2.6mmol/l. How low to lower LDL remains an open question. Preliminary evidence from the Post Coronary Artery Bypass Trial[4] suggests that lower is better but this was an angiographic rather than an event study. Ongoing studies such as TNT and SEARCH will provide more definitive information on this question. In the meantime it is the clinical practice of the author to lower LDL cholesterol if possible to <2.5mmol/l.

References

1 Scandinavian Simvastatin Survival Study Group. Randomised trial of cholesterol lowering in 4444 patients with coronary heart disease. The Scandinavian simvastatin survival study. *Lancet* 1994; **344**: 1383–9.
2 Sacks FM, Pfeffer MA, Moye LA *et al*. The effect of pravastatin on coronary events after myocardial infarction in patients with average cholesterol levels. *N Engl J Med* 1996; **335**: 1001–9.
3 The Long-Term Intervention with Pravastatin in Ischaemic Disease (LIPID) Study Group. Prevention of cardiovascular events and death with pravastatin in patients with coronary heart disease and a broad range of initial cholesterol levels. *N Engl J Med* 1998; **339**: 1349–57.

4 Post Coronary Artery Bypass Trial Investigators. The effect of aggressive lowering of low density lipoprotein cholesterol levels and low dose anticoagulation on obstructive changes in saphenous vein bypass grafts. *N Engl J Med* 1997; **336**: 153–62.

11 What drugs should I choose to treat dyslipidaemia, and how should I monitor treatment?

John Betteridge

Statins inhibit the conversion of HMG-CoA to mevalonate (the rate-determining step in cholesterol synthesis). Hepatic LDL receptors (recognising both apoproteins E and B) are upregulated, and uptake of LDL cholesterol and remnant particles (IDL) is increased. Hepatic VLDL output is also modestly decreased. Plasma LDL-cholesterol levels thus fall by 30–60% with the bulk of the decrease with the starting dose. A further 7% LDL reduction is obtained for each doubling of the dose. HDL cholesterol levels are modestly reduced ($\approx$8%), and if plasma triglyceride levels are above 2.5mmol/l, these are lowered by a similar fraction as LDL.

Statins are the first choice for patients requiring LDL reduction, and for treatment of mixed lipaemia if triglycerides are below 5mmol/l. Action on hepatic VLDL output probably underlies the modest reduction in cholesterol levels in patients homozygous for receptor negative familial hypercholesterolaemia (FH). There is little information on the use of statins in children, and they should be stopped in women at least 6 weeks prior to conception.

Anion-exchange resins interrupt the enterohepatic circulation of bile and cholesterol, causing body levels to fall. Hepatic LDL activity is upregulated to obtain cholesterol for new bile acid formation. LDL reductions of up to 30% can be achieved. They may increase triglyceride levels to a modest and often transient degree. Their poor tolerability generally reserves them for use in children heterozygous for FH, the treatment (in combination with statins) of severe adult FH, in FH women contemplating pregnancy (when some physicians use them in preference to statins) and in patients intolerant of statins. The resins have been used with positive outcome in several angiographic trials and in an early positive end point trial (the Lipid Research Clinics trial).

Fibrates are ligands for the nuclear hormone receptors, peroxisome proliferation activator receptors (PPARs). They decrease apoprotein C-III synthesis (an inhibitor of lipoprotein lipase) and therefore increase lipoprotein lipase activity. Triglyceride levels thus fall by 40–60%. They also upregulate apoprotein A-1 synthesis (the major protein of HDL). HDL cholesterol levels rise by 10–20%. Fibrates also lower LDL cholesterol in primary hyper-cholesterolaemia (type IIa hyperlipidaemia) by 15–25%. They are first line treatment for severe hypertriglyceridaemia and (in combination with statins) in severe mixed lipaemia. They are second line drugs in patients intolerant of statins for hyper-cholesterolaemia and mixed lipaemia. Data from end point clinical trials are not extensive and concerns over fibrate safety have remained since the original WHO clofibrate trial which was asso-ciated with increased non-CHD deaths. However the Helsinki Heart Study showed a positive outcome and the recent VA HIT trial, again with gemfibrozil, was positive. However the recent secondary BIP prevention study with bezafibrate was negative.

High dose fish oil capsules have a role in the treatment of severe hypertriglyceridaemia. They reduce hepatic VLDL output. In practice they are used in combination with fibrates and occasionally statins. The author has also used them in rare patients with familial hypertriglyceridaemia during pregnancy to protect against pancreatitis.

Further reading
Betteridge DJ, Morrell JM. *Clinicians' guide to lipids and coronary heart disease.* London: Chapman & Hall Medical, 1998.
Betteridge DJ, Illingworth DR, Shepherd J, eds. *Lipoproteins in health and disease.* London: Edward Arnold, 1999.

12 What are the side effects of lipid-lowering therapy, and how should they be monitored?

John Betteridge

Statins

These are generally well tolerated. In the major end point trials, adverse events were little different from placebo.

- *Myositis,* defined as painful, tender muscles with a high CPK, is rare, occurring with a frequency of lower than 1 in 10,000 patient years. Routine CPK measurement is not recommended as modest elevations (generally secondary to physical activity) are quite common even in patients on placebo treatment. It is important to remember that black patients have higher CPKs than whites, and that hypothyroidism is an important cause of raised CPK. Patients should be warned to stop the drugs if severe muscle pain is experienced.
- *Liver function* should be checked prior to statin therapy as abnormal hepatic function and high alcohol intake are relative contraindications for these drugs which are metabolised principally through the liver. Approximately one in 400 patients will develop greater than 3-fold transaminase increases which revert to normal with dose reduction or stopping of the drug. They can be used in moderate renal impairment. It is good practice to check liver function tests periodically during statin therapy.

Fibrates

These are also generally well tolerated but can also cause myositis and hepatic dysfunction. Clofibrate (in the WHO trial) was associated with increased gallstone formation through increased biliary cholesterol content. This drug is now redundant and the newer fibrates have less impact on biliary composition. Doubt remains concerning long term safety with the fibrate class in terms of non-cardiac mortality. However the WHO clofibrate trial was the major contributor to this concern. The recent VA HIT study (reported at the AHA meeting in Dallas, November 1998) showed that gemfibrozil reduced risk by approximately a quarter in post-MI men with average LDL but low HDL cholesterol concentrations with no increase in non-CHD adverse events.

Drug interactions

Care should be exercised when statins are combined with fibrates or used in patients taking cyclosporin (e.g. transplant patients) as the risk of side effects (particularly myositis) is increased. Dosage should be limited in transplant patients taking cyclosporin as drug levels are increased. Care should also be exercised when used in combination with drugs metabolised through the cytochrome P450 pathway (e.g. antifungals, erythromycin) as there is a potential for interactions. There is a theoretical potential for interaction with warfarin but the author has not found this a problem in practice.

Resins

The resins are associated with a high frequency of gastrointestinal side effects which limit their use. They may interfere with the absorption of other drugs so should be taken either one hour before or four hours after other therapeutic agents. The resins theoretically may interfere with the absorption of fat soluble vitamins and folic acid but this is not a major problem in practice. However, perhaps with increasing indication of the role of homo-cysteine as a risk factor, folic acid supplements might be recommended in patients on resins.

13 Is there a role for prescribing antioxidant vitamins to patients with coronary artery disease? If so, who should get them, and at what dose?

Peter Clifton

Three large prospective studies have shown that vitamin E users have a 40% lower rate of coronary artery disease. At least 100 IU/day of supplement is required to gain benefit. However, one large study in postmenopausal women showed no benefit from vitamin E supplementation, but high dietary vitamin E consumption reduced the risk by 58%.

At present there are only two intervention studies in patients with coronary artery disease available to guide therapeutic decisions. The CHAOS study[1] used 400 or 800 IU/day while the ATBC study[2] used 50 IU/day. Both studies showed that vitamin E does not save lives in patients with coronary artery disease and that it may increase the number of deaths. Both studies also agree that non-fatal myocardial infarctions are reduced significantly, by 38% in the ATBC study and by 77% in the CHAOS study, with a 53% reduction in combined events in the latter study. In the CHAOS study of 2002 patients, 27 heart attacks were prevented at the expense of 9 additional deaths (albeit statistically non-significant) while in the ATBC study the 15 fewer non-fatal heart attacks were balanced by 15 additional cardiovascular deaths. In the latter study it could be argued that the low dose of vitamin E used did not prevent myocardial infarction but when one occurred it was more often fatal. Until more compelling evidence is available the potential adverse effect of vitamin E does not outweigh the benefit of fewer non-fatal myocardial infarctions. Patients should be advised to eat diets rich in fruit and vegetables instead.

References

1 Stephens NG, Parsons A, Schofield PM *et al*. Randomised controlled trial of vitamin E in patients with coronary disease: Cambridge Heart Antioxidant Study. *Lancet* 1996;**347**: 781–6.

2 Rapola JM, Virtamo J, Ripatti S *et al*. Randomised trial of alpha-tocopherol and beta-carotene supplements on incidence of major coronary events in men with previous myocardial infarction. *Lancet* 1997;**349**: 1715–20.

14 What is the sensitivity, specificity and positive predictive value of an abnormal exercise test?

Vic Froelicher

While sensitivity (% of those with disease who have an abnormal test) and specificity (% of those without disease who have a normal test) are relatively independent of disease prevalence they are reciprocally related and dependent upon the cut point or criterion chosen for diagnosis. The positive predictive value of an abnormal test (% of those with an abnormal test that have disease) is directly related to the prevalence of disease. Another way to compare the diagnostic characteristics of a test is by use of predictive accuracy that is the percentage of total true calls (both negative and positive). While it is affected by disease prevalence, since diagnostic testing is usually only indicated when the pre-test probability is 50% (i.e. a disease prevalence of 50%) this measurement is a simple way of comparing test performance.

Meta-analysis of the exercise test studies with angiographic correlates has demonstrated the standard ST response (1mm depression) to have an average sensitivity of 68% and a specificity of 72% and a predictive accuracy of 69%.[1] But most of these studies have been affected by work up bias that means that those with abnormal tests were more likely to be entered into the studies to be catheterised. When work up bias is removed by having all patients with chest pain undergo catheterisation different results are obtained though the predictive accuracy remains the same. In such a study we found a sensitivity of 45% and a specificity of 85%.[2] It appears that this is how the test performs in the clinic or doctor's office. However, the inclusion of clinical and other test results in scores can increase the predictive accuracy of the standard exercise test to nearly 90%.[3]

References

1 Gianrossi R, Detrano R, Mulvihill D *et al*. Exercise-induced ST depression in the diagnosis of coronary artery disease: a meta-analysis. *Circulation* 1989;**80**: 87–98.

2 Froelicher VF, Lehmann KG, Thomas R *et al*. The ECG exercise test in a population with reduced workup bias: diagnostic performance, computerized interpretation, and multivariable prediction. Veterans

Affairs Cooperative Study in Health Services #016 (QUEXTA) Study Group. Quantitative exercise testing and angiography. *Ann Intern Med* 1998;**128**: 965–74.

3 Do D, West JA, Morise A *et al.* A consensus approach to diagnosing coronary artery disease based on clinical and exercise test data. *Chest* 1997;**111**: 1742–9.

15 What are the risks of exercise testing? What are the contraindications?

Joseph F Malouf

Although exercise testing is generally considered a safe procedure, acute myocardial infarction and death have been reported (up to 10 per 10,000 tests performed in some studies). The risk is greater in the post-MI patient and in those being evaluated for malignant ventricular arrhythmias. The rate of sudden cardiac death during exercise has ranged from zero to as high as 5% per 100,000 tests performed. Guidelines for exercise testing for North America have now been made available.[1] Table 15.1 lists absolute and relative contraindications to exercise testing. In patients recovering from acute myocardial infarction, a low level exercise test before discharge helps identify those patients at high risk for future cardiac events. In addition to being a source of reassurance to the patient and his/her family, the test may also provide guidelines for an exercise programme and resumption of work and normal sexual activities.

The sensitivity ranges from a low of 40% for single vessel coronary artery disease to up to 90% for angiographically severe three vessel disease, with a mean sensitivity of 66%. The specificity of the test is ~85% when at least 0.1mV horizontal or downsloping ST-segment depression are used as markers of ischaemia. In patients with a positive exercise test, an ischaemic threshold less than 70% of the patient's age predicted maximum heart rate is indicative of severe disease.

Various drugs may affect interpretation of the exercise test either because of haemodynamic alterations in the myocardial response to exercise or because the drug has direct electro-physiologic effects that can affect the interpretation of the electro-cardiogram. The decision to stop medications prior to an exercise test depends on the drug and the reasons for using it. Some institutions withhold beta blockers for 48 hours prior to exercise testing if there is doubt about the diagnosis of coronary artery disease.

Table 15.1   Absolute and relative contraindications to exercise testing*

Absolute

Acute myocardial infarction (within 3 to 5 days)

Unstable angina

Uncontrolled cardiac arrhythmias causing symptoms of haemodynamic compromise

Active endocarditis

Symptomatic severe aortic stenosis

Uncontrolled symptomatic heart failure

Acute pulmonary embolus or pulmonary infarction

Acute non-cardiac disorder that may affect exercise performance or be aggravated by exercise (e.g. infection, renal failure, thyrotoxicosis)

Acute myocarditis or pericarditis

Physical disability that would preclude safe and adequate test performance

Thrombosis of lower extremity

Relative

Left main coronary stenosis or its equivalent

Moderate stenotic valvular heart disease

Electrolyte abnormalities

Significant arterial or pulmonary hypertension

Tachyarrhythmias or bradyarrhythmias

Hypertrophic cardiomyopathy

Mental impairment leading to inability to cooperate

High degree atrioventricular block

*Relative contraindications can be superseded if benefits outweigh risks of exercise.

From Fletcher GF, Balady G, Froelicher VF *et al.* Exercise standards: a statement for Healthcare Professionals from the American Heart Association Writing Group. *Circulation* 1995;**9**: 580–615. (Reproduced by permission.)

References

1. Gibbons RJ, Chatterjee K, Daley J *et al.* ACC/AHA/ACP-ASIM guidelines for the management of patients with chronic stable angina: a report of the American College of Cardiology/American Heart Association Task Force on Practice Guidelines. *J Am Coll Cardiol* 1999;**33**: 2092–197.

16 What are the stratification data for risk from exercise tests in patients with angina? Which patterns of response warrant referral for angiography?

Vic Froelicher

The best evidence available on these questions is found in the two studies that used the appropriate statistical techniques to find the risk markers that were independently and statistically associated with the time to cardiovascular events. Both studies were performed in large populations (>3000 patients with probable coronary disease) and had five year follow-up. The Veteran's Affairs (VA) study was performed only in men and the risk factors identified were a history of congestive heart failure (CHF) or digoxin administration, an abnormal systolic blood pressure (SBP) response, limitation in exercise capacity, and ST depression.[1] The DUKE study included both genders and has been reproduced in the VA as well as other populations.[2] It includes exercise capacity, ST depression and whether or not angina occurred. The DUKE score has been included in all of the major guidelines in the form of a nomogram that calculates the estimated annual mortality due to cardiovascular events.

In general, an estimate more than 1 or 2% is high risk and should lead to a cardiac catheterisation that provides the "road map" for intervention. Certainly a clinical history consistent with congestive heart failure raises the annual mortality of any patient with angina and this is not considered in the DUKE score. Exercise capacity has been a consistent predictor of prognosis and disease severity. This is best measured in METs (multiples of basal oxygen consumption). In clinical practice this has been estimated from treadmill speed and grade but future studies may show the actual analysis of expired gases to be more accurate. Numerous studies have attempted to use equations to predict severe angiographic disease rather than prognosis but these have not been as well validated.[3]

References

1 Morrow K, Morris CK, Froelicher VF *et al.* Prediction of cardiovascular death in men undergoing noninvasive evaluation for CAD. *Ann Int Med* 1993;**118**: 689–95.

2 Marks D, Shaw L, Harrell FE Jr *et al.* Prognostic value of a treadmill exercise score in outpatients with suspected coronary artery disease. *N Engl J Med* 1991;**325**: 849–53.

3 Do D, West JA, Morise A *et al.* Agreement in predicting severe angiographic coronary artery disease using clinical and exercise test data. *Am Heart J* 1997;**134**: 672–9.

17 Who should have a thallium scan? How does it compare with standard exercise tests in determining risk ?

Liz Prvulovich

Exercise electrocardiography (ECG) is often the initial test in patients with chest pain being investigated for coronary artery disease (CAD). When this is unhelpful or leaves doubt then myocardial perfusion imaging (MPI) is recommended. This may occur when equivocal ST segment changes occur with exercise, the exercise ECG is abnormal in a patient at low risk for CAD or normal in a patient at high risk. MPI should be used instead of exercise ECG when a patient has restricted exercise tolerance and when the resting ECG is abnormal.[1] Importantly, recent data confirm that investigative strategies for chest pain which include MPI are cost effective.[2]

The prognostic value of MPI arises from the relationship between the depth and extent of perfusion abnormalities and the likelihood of future cardiac events. A normal MPI scan after adequate stress predicts a favourable prognosis (cardiac event rate below 1% annually).[3] Conversely, severe and extensive inducible perfusion defects imply a poor prognosis, as do stress-induced left ventricular dilatation and increased lung uptake of tracer. Several studies have shown that MPI is the most powerful single prognostic test and that it provides independent and incremental information to the exercise ECG in nearly all settings.[3,4] A prognostic strategy including MPI is also cost effective.[5]

References
1 Underwood SR, Godman B, Salyani S *et al.* Economics of myocardial perfusion imaging in Europe – The Empire Study. *Eur Heart J* 1999;**20**: 157–66.
2 De Bono D, for the joint working party of the British Cardiac Society and Royal College of Physicians of London. Investigation and management of stable angina: revised guidelines. *Heart* 1999;**81**: 546–55.
3 Brown KA. Prognostic value of myocardial perfusion imaging: state of the art and new developments. *J Nucl Cardiol* 1996;**3**: 516–38.
4 Ladenheim ML, Kotler TS, Pollock BH *et al.* Incremental prognostic power of clinical history, exercise electrocardiography and myocardial perfusion scintigraphy in patients with suspected coronary disease. *Am J Cardiol* 1987;**59**: 270–7.

5 Hachamavitch R, Berman DS, Shaw LJ *et al.* Incremental prognostic value of myocardial perfusion single photon emission computed tomography for the prediction of cardiac death; differential stratification for the risk of cardiac death and myocardial infarction. *Circulation* 1998;**97**: 535–43.

18 What are hibernating and stunned myocardium? What echocardiographic techniques are useful for detecting them? How do these methods compare with others available?

Petros Nihoyannopoulos

The physiologic abnormalities that are associated with resting myocardial dysfunction and viable myocardium range from reduced resting myocardial flow and preserved metabolic uptake of ^{18}F-2-Deoxyglucose (FDG) (**hibernating myocardium**) to patients in whom resting myocardial flow is preserved (**stunned myocardium**). Animal studies[1] suggest that stunning may progress to hibernation as part of an adaptive response. As coronary flow reserve decreases, fasting FDG uptake increases while resting flow remains normal (chronic stunning). Later on, during continuing ischaemia, flow is reduced while FDG uptake continues, characteristic of hibernation.

Assessing myocardial viability is important in coronary artery disease patients with ventricular dysfunction because its presence improves left ventricular function and survival following revascularisation.[2,3] Diagnostic methods include **positron emission tomography (PET)**, based on the detection of metabolic activity, ^{201}**Tl single-photon emission computed tomography (Tl-SPECT)**, to assess cell membrane integrity by rest/redistribution and the assessment of contractile reserve by **dobutamine stress echocardiography**. Echocardiography can assess the presence of myocardial viability by looking at contractile reserve following inotropic stimulation with dobutamine (dobutamine stress echocardiography). This differentiates viable myocardium (presence of contractile reserve) from non-viable scarred myocardium (absence of contractile reserve) in patients with ventricular dysfunction at rest. More recently, **myocardial contrast echocardiography (MCE)** has been proposed as a method to assess myocardial perfusion and viability. Myocardial opacification produced by the presence of microbubbles in the coronary microcirculation has been considered synonymous with preserved microvascular integrity.

Using detailed histology from explanted hearts in patients undergoing heart transplantation, Baumgartner *et al.* compared PET, SPECT and echo to detect viable myocardium[4]. While segments with >50% of viable myocytes were equally well predicted by all three non-invasive tests, in segments with <50% of viable myocytes the response to dobutamine was poor in relation to SPECT and PET, which showed equal sensitivities. However, taking survival as an end point, patients with at least 42% of viable segments during dobutamine stress echocardiography had a better long term survival following revascularisation.[3]

References

1 Fallavollita JA, Canty JM. Differential ^{18}F-2-Deoxyglucose uptake in viable dysfunctional myocardium with normal resting perfusion. *Circulation* 1999;**99**: 2798–805.

2 Di Carli MF, Asgrzadie F, Schelbert H *et al.* Quantitative relation between myocardial viability and improvement in heart failure symptoms after revascularisation in patients with ischaemic cardiomyopathy. *Circulation* 1995;**92**: 3436–44.

3 Senior R, Kaul S, Lahiri A. Myocardial viability on echocardiography predicts long-term survival after revascularisation in patients with ischaemic congestive heart failure. *J Am Coll Cardiol* 1999;**33**: 1848–54.

4 Baumgartner H, Porenta G, Lau Y-K *et al.* Assessment of myocardial viability by dobutamine echocardiography, positron emission tomography and thallium-201 SPECT. *J Am Coll Cardiol* 1998;**32**: 1701–8.

19 Which class of antianginal agent should I prescribe in stable angina? Does it matter?

Henry Purcell

Nitrates

All patients with angina pectoris should have sublingual glyceryl trinitrate (GTN) for the rapid relief of acute pain. Long-acting isosorbide dinitrate (ISDN) and isosorbide mononitrate (ISMN) preparations are also available but have not been shown to influence mortality in post-myocardial infarction (MI) patients.

Beta blockers

In the absence of contraindications, beta blockers are preferred as initial therapy for angina.[1] Evidence for this is strongest for patients with prior MI. Long term trials show that there is a 23% reduction in the odds of death among MI survivors randomised to beta blockers.[2]

Calcium antagonists

Calcium antagonists (especially those which reduce heart rate) are suitable as initial therapy when beta blockers are contra-indicated or poorly tolerated. Outcome trials are underway but there is currently little evidence to suggest they improve prognosis post-MI, although diltiazem and verapamil may reduce the risk of reinfarction in patients without heart failure,[3] and amlodipine may benefit certain patients with heart failure.

Other agents

Nicorandil, a potassium channel opener with a nitrate moiety, and the metabolic agent, trimetazidine, may also be useful, but these have not been tested in outcome studies.

Many patients with exertional symptoms may need a combination of anti-anginals, but there is little evidence to support the use of "triple therapy". Patients requiring this should be assessed for revascularisation. There are no important differences in the effectiveness of the principal classes of anti-anginal used singly or in combination. Choices should be based on those producing fewest side effects, good compliance and cost effectiveness.[4]

References

1 ACC/AHA/ACP-ASIM Guidelines for the management of patients with chronic stable angina: executive summary and recommendations. *Circulation* 1999;**99**: 2829–48.
2 Freemantle N, Cleland J, Young P *et al.* β blockade after myocardial infarction: systematic review and meta regression analysis. *BMJ* 1999;**318**: 1730–7.
3 Task Force of the European Society of Cardiology. Management of stable angina pectoris. *Eur Heart J* 1997;**18**: 394–413.
4 Petticrew M, Sculpher M, Kelland J *et al.* Effective management of stable angina. *Qual Health Care* 1998;**7**: 109–16.

20 What is the role of troponin T in the diagnosis and risk stratification of acute coronary syndromes?

David J Brull

A significant proportion of patients presenting to accident and emergency departments complain of chest pain. Early risk stratification is vital with the primary aim being to identify life-threatening conditions such as acute coronary syndromes (ACS) and ensure their appropriate management, especially since the majority of patients have either non-cardiac chest pain or stable angina and are at low risk.

Standard diagnostic approach

The standard approach to the diagnosis of acute chest pain is to combine features of the clinical history, including cardiac risk factor profile, with electrocardiogaphic features and biochemical markers. The Braunwald classification was initially introduced to allow the identification of patients with unstable angina at different levels of risk. It correlates well with in-hospital event rate and prognosis. Unfortunately symptoms may be difficult to interpret and clinical assessment alone is insufficient for risk stratification. Many studies have shown that admission 12-lead ECG provides direct prognostic information in patients with ACS. However, as many as 50% of patients ultimately diagnosed as having either unstable angina or myocardial infarction present with either a normal ECG or with minor or non-specific ECG changes only.

Traditionally the biochemical diagnosis of myocardial injury was confirmed by measurements of non-specific enzymes such as CK-MB mass or myoglobin, whose levels may also be elevated after non-cardiac injury. The availability of rapid and accurate bedside assays of cardiac troponin T has transformed the diagnostic process. Troponin T is an essential structural protein of the myocardial sarcomere. It is a highly sensitive and specific marker of myocardial damage that is not detectable in the healthy state. Troponin T is released within 4–6 hours of injury peaking after 12 to 24 hours. Elevated levels of troponin T reflect even minor myocardial damage and remain detectable for up to 14 days. An elevated troponin T has a predictive value for myocardial ischaemia several times higher than CK-MB mass.

Troponin T as a diagnostic tool

Troponin T can be used both as a diagnostic and a prognostic tool in the Accident and Emergency Department. Repeated troponin assays taken 4–6 hours apart have been used to successfully identify all patients with MI even in the absence of ST elevation.[1] Individuals who were troponin T negative were shown to be at low short term risk. Troponin T accurately reflects the degree of myocardial necrosis with the overall risk of death following an ACS being directly related to the levels detected. Data from the Fragmin During Instability in Coronary Artery Disease trial (FRISC) demonstrated that patients with the highest levels of troponin T following an ACS carried the highest risk of death and MI, in contrast to those who were troponin T negative who were at low risk.[2] A subset from the GUSTO IIa trial had similar findings for non-ST elevation ACS where troponin T positive patients had a much higher risk of death and heart failure than troponin T negative individuals.[3]

Risk stratification

The initial step in risk stratification is an ECG. Patients with acute ST elevation are considered to have an acute MI and require reperfusion therapy according to local protocols. Individuals with ST depression are also at high risk and require admission for further evaluation. The presence of a positive troponin T in this group further confirms them as high risk. In situations where patients present either with a normal ECG or with T wave changes only, the value of a positive troponin T is vital in risk stratification. All patients who are troponin T positive should be considered as high risk, whilst in contrast, a negative troponin T 12 hours or more after the onset of symptoms puts the individual in a low risk group. If the result of a negative troponin T test taken 12 hours or more after the onset of chest pain is taken in conjunction with a pre-discharge exercise test, this further reduces the chance of an inappropriate discharge.[4] Figure 20.1 illustrates one possible management algorithm.

Figure 20.1   Risk stratification algorithm for acute chest pain

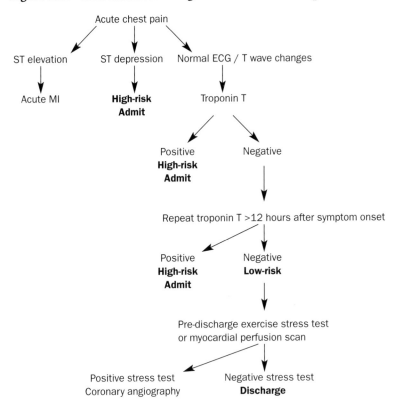

Conclusion

Troponin T has a vital role in the triage of patients presenting with chest pain. A positive test identifies high-risk individuals who may benefit from aggressive anti-platelet therapy or early intervention, whilst negative troponin T tests 12 or more hours after the onset of symptoms identify those at low risk who can be considered for early hospital discharge.

References

1 Hamm CW, Goldmann BU, Heeschen C *et al*. Emergency room triage of patients with acute chest pain by means of rapid testing for cardiac troponin T or troponin I. *N Engl J Med* 1997; **337**: 1648–53.
2 Lindahl B, Venge P, Wallentin L, for the FRISC Study Group. Relation between troponin T and the risk of subsequent cardiac events in unstable coronary artery disease. Circulation 1996;**93**: 1651–57.
3 Ohman EM, Armstrong PW, Christensen RH *et al*. for the GUSTO IIa Investigators. Cardiac troponin T levels for risk stratification in acute myocardial ischemia. *N Engl J Med* 1996;**335**: 1333–41.
4 Lindahl B, Andren B, Ohlsson J *et al*. Risk stratification in unstable coronary artery disease. Additive value of troponin T determinations and pre-discharge exercise tests. *Eur Heart J* 1997;**18**: 762–70.

21 What are the risks of myocardial infarction and death in someone with unstable angina during hospital admission, at six months and one year?

Diana Holdright

The risks of myocardial infarction (MI) and death following the diagnosis of unstable angina (UA) depend on the accuracy of the diagnosis. Braunwald's classification categorises patients according to the severity of the pain (new onset/accelerated and pain at rest, either within the last 48 hours or >48 hours) and to the clinical circumstances (primary, secondary (e.g. to anaemia) and post-infarction). Using this classification, one study showed an in-hospital AMI/death rate of 11% for patients with rest pain within the last 48 hours, 4% for patients with rest pain >48 hours previously and 4% for patients with new onset/accelerated angina.[1] The in-hospital AMI/death rate was markedly raised in patients with post-infarct angina (46%) compared with patients with "primary" unstable angina.

The event rate is highest at and shortly following presentation, falling off rapidly in the first few months to a level similar to stable angina patients after one year. Patients with new onset angina have a better prognosis than those with acceleration of previously stable angina or patients with rest pain. Patients with accelerated or crescendo angina have an in-hospital mortality of 2-8% and a 1 year survival of 90%. Although patients with non-Q wave MI, also considered within the umbrella term UA, have a more benign in-hospital course than Q-wave MI patients, they have higher readmission, reinfarction and revascularisation rates subsequently. Infarct extension in-hospital is associated with a far worse prognosis in non-Q wave MI (43% mortality, vs 15% in Q wave MI). The following are also associated with a worse prognosis in unstable angina: ST segment deviation on the ECG (but not T wave changes), elevated cardiac enzymes, transient myocardial ischaemia on Holter monitoring, an abnormal pre-discharge exercise test, extensive coronary artery disease and impaired left ventricular function.

The OASIS registry,[2] gave 7 day death/MI rates of 3.7–5.6% and 6 month rates of 8.8–11.9%. Similarly, the VANQWISH trial[3] gave the following rates of death/non-fatal MI: 3.2–7% at hospital discharge, 5.7–10.3% at 1 month and 18.6–24% at 1 year.

References

1 Van Miltenburg AJ, Simoons ML, Veerhoek RJ *et al.* Incidence and follow-up of Braunwald subgroups in unstable angina pectoris. *J Am Coll Cardiol* 1995;**25**: 1286–92.

2 Yusuf S, Flather M, Pogue J *et al.* for the OASIS (Organisation to Assess Strategies for Ischaemic Syndromes) Registry Investigators. Variations between countries in invasive cardiac procedures and outcomes in patients with suspected unstable angina or myocardial infarction without initial ST elevation. *Lancet* 1998;**352**: 507–14.

3 Boden WE, O'Rourke RA, Crawford MH *et al.* for the Veterans Affairs Non-Q Wave Infarction Strategies in Hospital (VANQWISH) Trial Investigators. Outcomes in patients with acute non-Q-wave myocardial infarction randomly assigned to an invasive as compared with a conservative management strategy. *N Engl J Med* 1998;**338**: 1785–92.

22 What medical treatments of unstable angina are of proven benefit?

Diana Holdright

The treatment of unstable angina is dictated by the underlying pathophysiology, namely, rupturing of an atheromatous plaque and secondary platelet aggregation, vasoconstriction and thrombus formation.

Anti-ischaemic therapy

Nitrates relieve ischaemic pain but there is no evidence of prognostic benefit from their use.

Calcium antagonists are effective anti-ischaemic and vasodilator drugs. However, in the absence of beta blockade, nifedipine should be avoided due to reflex tachycardia. Verapamil and diltiazem have useful rate-lowering properties, but should be used cautiously in patients with ventricular dysfunction and patients already taking beta blockers.

Beta-adrenoceptor blockers are an important treatment in unstable angina, not only relieving symptoms but also reducing the likelihood of progression to infarction and cardiac death. There is no evidence to favour one class of beta blocker over another.

Antithrombotic therapy

Aspirin has an important and undisputed role in the treatment of unstable angina, reducing the risk of fatal/non-fatal MI by 70% acutely, by 60% at 3 months and by 52% at 2 years.[1] A first dose of 160-325mg should be followed by a maintenance dose of ≥75mg daily.

Ticlopidine and *clopidogrel*, antagonists of ADP-mediated platelet aggregation, are possible alternatives in patients unable to take aspirin, although ticlopidine has important side effects and trials using clopidogrel have yet to be completed (e.g. CURE study).

Glycoprotein IIb/IIIa inhibitors (e.g. abciximab, tirofiban and eptifibatide) are potent anti-platelet agents and are effective, but costly, in patients with unstable angina undergoing PTCA. More recent data support a wider role for their use in the medical management of high-risk patients with unstable angina i.e. recurrent ischaemia, raised troponia levels, haemodynamic instability, major arrhythmia and early post-infarction unstable angina.[2]

Unfractionated heparin reduces ischaemic episodes but most trials have not shown greater benefit from heparin and aspirin compared with aspirin alone. However, a meta-analysis gave a 7.9% incidence of death/MI with the combination compared with 10.4% with aspirin alone.[3]

Low molecular weight heparins (e.g. dalteparin, enoxaparin) are at least as effective as heparin and are tending to replace heparin as standard therapy.[4]

Thrombolytics are of no proven benefit and should be avoided.

References
1. Theroux P, Fuster V. Acute coronary syndromes. *Circulation* 1998;**97**: 1195–206.
2. National Institute for Clinical Excellence. *Guidance on the use of glycoprotein IIb/IIIa inhibitors in the treatment of acute coronary syndromes.* Technology Appraisal Guidance-No. 12, September 2000. (www.nice.org.uk)
3 Oler A, Whooley MA, Oler J. Grady D. Adding heparin to aspirin reduces the incidence of myocardial infarction and death in patients with unstable angina. *JAMA* 1996;**276**: 811–15.
4 Cohen M, Demers C, Gurfinkel EP *et al.* A comparison of low-molecular weight heparin with unfractionated heparin for unstable coronary artery disease: Efficiency and Safety of Subcutaneous Enoxaparin in Non-Q-Wave Coronary Events (ESSENCE) Study Group. *N Engl J Med*; 1997;**337**: 447–52.

23 Under what circumstances should the patient with unstable angina undergo PTCA or CABG?

Diana Holdright

Until recently, published trials and registry data comparing early invasive and conservative strategies in patients with unstable angina (UA) and non-Q wave myocardial infarction (NQMI) suggested no overall benefit from an early invasive approach. Indeed, there was the impression that patients fared better with an initial conservative approach. However, the most recently published trial (FRISC II),[1] reflecting modern interventional practice, new stent technology and adjunctive medical therapies (e.g. the glycoprotein IIb/IIIa antagonists) together with improved bypass and myocardial preservation techniques and greater use of arterial conduits has shown significant mortality and morbidity benefit from an early invasive approach.

The first trial to assess these two management strategies, TIMI IIIB, randomised patients with UA/NQMI to angiography within 24–48 hours followed by PTCA/CABG if appropriate.[2] The primary end point of death/MI/positive treadmill test at 6 weeks was 18.1% for the conservative strategy and 16.2% for the invasive strategy (p = NS). Death/MI occurred in 7.8% and 7.2% at 6 weeks (p = NS) and in 12.2% and 10.8% at 1 year (p = NS). However, 64% of patients crossed over to the invasive strategy because of recurrent angina or an abnormal treadmill test, raising doubts about the clinical application of the trial results.

The VANQWISH study similarly randomised patients with NQMI.[3] Death or non-fatal MI occurred in 7% (invasive) vs 3.2% (conservative, p = 0.004) at hospital discharge, in 10.3% vs 5.7% at 1 month (p = 0.0012) and in 24% vs 18.6% at 1 year (p = 0.05). However, with longer follow up (23 months) the mortality difference was lost. Of note, 9% of eligible patients were excluded due to very high-risk ischaemic complications. In contrast to TIMI IIIB, only 29% patients crossed over from the conservative arm.

The OASIS registry highlighted different management strategies for UA by country.[4] Angiography rates varied from 2% (Poland) to 58% (US) and 60% (Brazil) at 7 days. Rates of PTCA and CABG by 7 days were highest in the US and Brazil (15.9% and 11.7%) and lowest in Canada/Australia/Hungary/Poland (5% and 1.6%). However, MI and death rates were similar for all countries during a 6 month follow up. Countries with high intervention rates had higher stroke rates but lower rates of recurrent angina and readmission for unstable angina.

The FRISC II study,[1] comparing early invasive and conservative strategies, together with the effect of placebo-controlled long term low molecular weight heparin (dalteparin), showed a reduction in death and myocardial infarction in the invasive group (9.4% vs 12.1% in the non-invasive group at 6 months, p = 0.031). Symptoms of angina and readmission were also halved by the invasive strategy. The greatest benefit was seen in high risk patients, in whom potentially beneficial treatments are often denied in routine clinical practice. By 6 months, 37% of the non-invasive group had crossed over to the invasive strategy. Although there was a higher event rate initially in the invasive group, associated with revascularisation, the event rate subsequently fell and the hazard curves crossed after 4 weeks. Thereafter, the event rate was consistently lower in the invasive group. Invasive treatment provided the greatest advantages in older patients, men, patients with a longer duration of angina, chest pain at rest and ST segment depression.

The favourable results of FRISC II reflect not only modern revascularisation technologies but probably also the intended delay prior to angiography and intervention. Patients in the invasive arm were initially stabilised medically, with the aim to perform all invasive procedures within seven days.

The consensus of opinion has thus changed and, where facilities permit, intensive medical therapy followed by angiography with a view to revascularisation is the preferred option for patients with unstable coronary artery disease.

References

1 Fragmin and Fast Revascularisation during InStability in Coronary artery disease (FRISC II) Investigators. Invasive compared with non-invasive treatment in unstable coronary-artery disease: FRISC II prospective randomised multicentre study. *Lancet* 1999;**354**: 708–15.

2 Anderson HV, Cannon CP, Stone PH *et al.* One-year results of the Thrombolysis in Myocardial Infarction (TIMI) IIIB clinical trial: a randomised comparison of tissue-type plasminogen activator versus placebo and early invasive versus early conservative strategies in unstable angina and non-Q wave myocardial infarction. *J Am Coll Cardiol* 1995;**26**: 1643–50.

3 Boden WE, O'Rourke RA, Crawford MH *et al.* for the Veterans Affairs Non-Q Wave Infarction Strategies in Hospital (VANQWISH) Trial

Investigators. Outcomes in patients with acute non-Q-wave myocardial infarction randomly assigned to an invasive as compared with a conservative management strategy. *N Engl J Med* 1998;**338**: 1785–1792.

4 Yusuf S, Flather M, Pogue J *et al.* for the OASIS (Organisation to Assess Strategies for Ischaemic Syndromes) Registry Investigators. Variations between countries in invasive cardiac procedures and outcomes in patients with suspected unstable angina or myocardial infarction without initial ST elevation. *Lancet* 1998;**352**: 507–14.

24 What new approaches are there to prevent restenosis following PTCA?

Richard Mansfield

Percutaneous transluminal coronary angioplasty (PTCA) is a well-established treatment for patients with coronary artery disease. However, the excellent initial procedural outcome is limited by the late development of restenosis occurring in approximately 30% of cases between 3 and 6 months. The introduction of intracoronary stents, which now account for more than 70% of all interventional procedures has had only a modest effect on restenosis rates. There were over 20,000 angioplasty or related procedures in the UK in 1996 and it is easy to appreciate the clinical and economic burden of restenosis.

Pharmacological approaches

To date no pharmacological agent has had a significant effect on reducing the incidence of restenosis. There are a number of reasons for this including the lack of correlation between animal models and the situation in man, the drug doses used or the power of some of the trials. Recent interest has focused on the use of antiproliferative agents such as paclitaxel and tranilast.

The antioxidant Probucol has been shown to be effective in limiting restenosis after balloon angioplasty. However, lack of licensing in some countries, limited data on the clinical impact of treatment, and the fact that pre-treatment for 4 weeks is required, may all be factors in limiting its use.

Gene therapy involves the transfer of DNA into host cells with the aim of inducing specific biological effects. Vectors for gene delivery include plasmid DNA-liposome complexes and viral vectors such as the replication deficient recombinant adenovirus. Design of appropriate delivery devices has taken a number of directions including double balloon catheters and perforated balloons allowing high pressure injection through radial pores. Various approaches have been used to limit experimental restenosis by inducing cell death (e.g. fas ligand gene to induce apoptosis), inhibiting smooth muscle cell migration (e.g. over-expression of TIMP-1 and eNOS) or by inhibiting cell cycle regulators of smooth muscle cell proliferation (e.g. antisense c-myc or c-myb oligonucleotides). There is a vast amount of experimental data, with early results from gene therapy trials for angiogenesis, but clinical trials for restenosis are awaited.

Brachytherapy

Over the last few years there has been considerable interest in intravascular brachytherapy (radiation therapy). The ability of ionising radiation to halt cell growth by damaging the DNA of dividing cells, and the view that neointimal hyperplasia represented a benign proliferative condition led to its application in vascular disease. A variety of catheter based delivery systems and radioactive stents are available using either beta (e.g. ^{32}P) or gamma (e.g. ^{192}Ir) sources. A number of studies have shown impressive results on reducing restenosis rates and many more are underway but enthusiasm for the technique should be tempered because there are concerns about long term safety. Indeed there are very recent reports of unexpected late thrombotic occlusion.

Photodynamic therapy (PTD) involves the local activation of a systemically administered photosensitising agent by non-ionising radiation in the form of non-thermal laser light. Many of the sensitising agents that have been studied have been products of porphyrin metabolism such as 5-aminolaevulinic acid. Much of the work in this field to date has been in the treatment of cancer but there is an accumulation of small and large animal data showing a reduction in neointimal hyperplasia after balloon injury. Favourable vessel wall remodelling has also been observed in a pig model of balloon coronary and iliac angioplasty. Reports of the clinical application of photodynamic therapy are limited but a clinical pilot study of adjuvant PDT in superficial femoral angioplasty showed it to be a safe and effective technique. Further work needs to be done to establish its role in coronary disease.

Further reading

Jenkins MP, Buonaccorsi GA *et al*. Reduction in the response to coronary and iliac artery injury with photodynamic therapy using 5-amino-laevulinic acid. *Cardiovasc Res* 2000;**45**: 478–85.

Kullo IJ, Simari RD, Schwartz RS. Vascular gene transfer; from bench to bedside. *Arterioscler Thromb Vasc Biol* 1999;**19**: 196–207.

Landzberg BR, Frishman WH, Lerrick K. Pathophysiology and pharmacological approaches for prevention of coronary artery restenosis following coronary artery balloon angioplasty and related procedures. *Prog Cardiovasc Dis* 1997;**34**: 361–98.

Weinberger J, Simon AD. Intracoronary irradiation for the prevention of restenosis. *Current Opin Cardiol* 1997;**12**: 468–74.

Yokoi H, Daida H, Kuwabara Y *et al.* Effectiveness of an antioxidant in preventing restenosis after percutaneous transluminal coronary angioplasty: the Probucol Angioplasty Restenosis Trial. *J Am Coll Cardiol* 1997;**30**: 855–62.

25 Which thrombolytics are currently available for treating acute myocardial infarction? Who should receive which one? What newer agents are there?

Anthony Gershlick

Thrombolysis

Natural thrombolysis occurs via the action of plasmin on fibrin thrombi. Plasmin is formed from plasminogen by cleavage of a single peptide bond. Plasmin is a non-specific protease and dissolves coagulation factors as well as fibrin clots. Three thrombolytic agents are currently available. Streptokinase (SK) forms a non-covalent link with plasminogen. The resultant conformational change exposes the active site on plasminogen to induce the formation of plasmin. Tissue plasminogen activator (tPA) is a serine protease and binds directly to fibrin via a lysine site, activating fibrin-bound plasminogen. The theoretical advantages of tPA are its increased specificity and potency because of its direct effect on fibrin-bound plasminogen. Being the product of recombinant DNA technology, there should be no allergic reaction to tPA. Unlike SK which should be used only once, tPA can be used repeatedly. Some, but not all, of these theoretical advantages translate into definite clinical benefit. Recently reteplase, a variation of tPA, has become available.

The Fibrinolytic Therapy Trialists Collaborative Group[1] summarised results from thrombolytic trials encompassing more than 100,000 patients. The overall relative risk reduction in 35 day mortality with treatment was 18% (p < 0.00001). The mortality at this time was ~13%, reduced to 8–9% with treatment. However, in real life where the population is older than in the trials the true mortality is about 18–20%. Administration of a thrombolytic saves about 30 lives in a 1000 in those presenting within 6 hours of symptom onset but only 20 lives in a 1000 when patients receive treatment between 6 and 12 hours after symptom onset. Aspirin has an independent beneficial effect on mortality and can be chewed.[2] The LATE Trial showed no benefit 12 hours after onset of symptoms.[3] Judging the onset of symptoms can be difficult and may be influenced by collateral flow from another artery. If a patient presents with stuttering symptoms over 24 hours or so but has had severe pain over a few hours and has an appropriately abnormal ECG, thrombolytic treatment should be seriously considered. Prehospital thrombolysis has been shown to reduce cardiac mortality compared to in-hospital thrombolysis by 17% (p = 0.03), by reducing the mean time to treatment by about one hour.[4] Despite this, prehospital thrombolysis has in general not been taken up for logistical reasons.

Is one thrombolytic better than another?

Although angiographic studies show higher early patency rates with tPA compared with SK (~70% vs ~35%), neither the GISSI-2 study[5] nor the ISIS-3 study found any difference in 30 day mortality rate (8.5% SK vs 8.9% tPA) and (10.6% for SK and 10.3% for tPA) respectively. In the GUSTO trial a more aggressive regimen was used, so called front-loaded tPA, producing a small but significant benefit favouring tPA (6.3% vs 7.3% p > 0.04). There were, however, an excess of strokes (0.72% for tPA vs 0.54% for SK). Combining deaths and strokes there was still a benefit favouring front-loaded tPA (6.9 % vs 7.8%).

Currently, in many countries streptokinase remains the first line treatment for AMI. This is because the advantage for tPA is modest and tPA is expensive ((£470) compared to SK (£80) per patient). Since streptokinase neutralising antibodies are formed from about day 4 onwards, tPA will need to be administered should the patient reinfarct after this time.

The lack of any large difference in clinical outcome between tPA and SK despite the difference in early angiographic patency needs to be explained. TPA is locally effective, with little systemic thrombolytic effect (for example on circulating plasminogen). It is, however, very specific, which is the cause for the excess in strokes. It has a short half life compared to SK. It has been clearly shown in animal models of arterial thrombotic occlusion that opening of the vessel by administration of tPA may be followed by early reocclusion, perhaps within minutes. The 90 minute angiogram cannot reflect the consequent reocclusion of the artery, which will happen less with SK which has a longer half life. Thus the increased patency with tPA may not translate into a decrease in mortality. The short half life of tPA means that heparin should be coadministered and continued for 24 hours although true benefit has never actually been proven.

What to give

Currently, the choice of thrombolytic varies by country and depends especially on the type of health care system and funding in place. In many countries, in the absence of previous administration the first line thrombolytic is SK (1.5 million units in 100 mls 5% dextrose/0.9% NaCl over 30–60 minutes). Alternatively, tPA is given as a 15mg bolus followed by 50mg over 60 minutes, then 35mg over a further 30 minutes. Based on the GUSTO study a case can be made for tPA in those presenting very early (<4 hours with large anterior infarcts). **New plasminogen activators** such as recombinant plasminogen activator (r-PA) and prourokinase are currently the subject of a number of clinical studies. **Reteplase (rPA)**, is a nonglycosylated deletion mutant of wild type tPA. It is the first member of the third generation thrombolytics, has a longer half life and is given as a double bolus (10IU + 10IU). Equivalence trials comparing tPA and reteplase have demonstrated no difference in outcome and currently these two drugs are interchangeable, with decisions about use being based on availability and price.[6] **Lanoteplase** has been withdrawn prior to launch because of patent issues and **TNK-tPA** is being trialled against tPA (ASSENT 2).[7] Bleeding with this new agent was between 2.8% and 7.4% dependent on dose (ASSENT 1).[8] Data suggest that there may be a role for "rescue" angioplasty in patients who fail to show electrocardiographic evidence of reperfusion.[9] However, results of randomised trials addressing this issue are awaited.

References

1 Fibrinolytic Therapy Trialists (FTT) Collaborative Group. Indications for fibrinolytic therapy in suspected acute myocardial infarction: collaborative overview of early mortality and major morbidity from all randomised trials of more than 1000 patients. *Lancet* 1994;**343**: 311–22.

2 Feldman M, Cryer B. Aspirin absorption rates and platelet inhibition times with 325mg buffered aspirin tablets (chewed or swallowed whole) and with buffered aspirin solution. *Am J Cardiol* 1999;**84**: 404–9.

3 LATE Study Group. Late assessment of thrombolytic efficiency (LATE) study with alteplase 6–24 hours after onset of acute myocardial infarction. *Lancet* 1993;**342**: 759–66.

4 The European Myocardial Infarction Project Group. Pre-hospital thrombolytic therapy in patients with suspected acute myocardial infarction. *N Engl J Med* 1993;**329**: 383–9.

5 GISSI-2. A factorial randomised trial of alteplase versus streptokinase and heparin versus no heparin among 12,490 patients with acute myocardial infarction. *Lancet* 1990;**336**: 65–71.

6 Hampton JR. The concept of equivalence and its application to the assessment of thrombolytic effects. *Eur Heart J* 1997;**18**: F22–7.

7 ASSENT Investigators. Single bolus tenecteplase compared with front-loaded alteplase in acute myocardial infarction: the ASSENT-2 double blind randomised trial. *Lancet* 1999;**354**: 716–22.

8 ASSENT-1 Investigators. Safety assessment of a single bolus administration of TNK-tissue plasminogen activator in AMI. *Am Heart J* 1999;**137**: 786–91.

9 Mukherjee D, Ellis SG. "Rescue" angioplasty for failed thrombolysis. *Cleve Clin J Med* 2000;**67**: 341–52.

26 Is angioplasty better than thrombolysis in myocardial infarction? Which patients should receive primary or "hot" angioplasty for these conditions?

Vincent S DeGeare and Cindy L Grines

In patients with ST elevation myocardial infarction (MI) there is impressive evidence that primary percutaneous transluminal coronary angioplasty (PTCA) results in lower morbidity and mortality than does intravenous thrombolysis. This was first demonstrated in the Primary Angioplasty in Myocardial Infarction (PAMI) trial where primary PTCA resulted in a significant reduction in in-hospital and 6 month composite of death plus non-fatal recurrent myocardial infarction.[1] There was also a significant reduction in intracranial bleeding with primary PTCA. The GUSTO IIb angioplasty substudy also showed a significant reduction in the combined end point of death, non-fatal reinfarction or disabling stroke at 30 days.[2] A recent meta-analysis of 10 trials comparing primary PTCA to intravenous thrombolytic therapy showed a 34% reduction in mortality (p = 0.02), a 65% reduction in total stroke (p = 0.007) and a 91% decrease in haemorrhagic stroke (p < 0.001) among patients undergoing primary PTCA.[3] In addition, PTCA has been shown to be superior to intravenous thrombolytic therapy in acute MI patients with cardiogenic shock, congestive heart failure,[4] prior coronary bypass surgery (where the culprit vessel is often a thrombosed saphenous vein graft) and in nearly all patients in whom thrombolytic therapy is contraindicated. However, data suggest that the success of primary intervention is dependent on the frequency with which the procedure is performed.[5] In addition, there are cost implications to providing such a service which, in any event, is unlikely to become available in every Western hospital.

References

1 Grines CL, Browne KF, Marco J *et al.* for the Primary Angioplasty in Myocardial Infarction Study Group. A comparison of immediate angioplasty with thrombolytic therapy for acute myocardial infarction. *N Engl J Med* 1993;**328**: 673–9.

2 The Global Use of Strategies to Open Occluded Coronary Arteries in Acute Coronary Syndromes (GUSTO IIb) Angioplasty substudy Investigators. A clinical trial comparing primary coronary angioplasty with tissue plasminogen activator for acute myocordial infarction. *N Engl J Med* 1997;**336**: 1621–8.

3 Weaver WD, Simes RJ, Betriu A, *et al.* Comparison of primary coronary angioplasty and intravenous thrombolytic therapy for acute myocardial infarction: a quantitative review. *JAMA* 1997;**278**: 2093–8.

4 Bates ER, Topol EJ. Limitations of thrombolytic therapy for acute myocardial infarction complicated by congestive heart failure and cardiogenic shock. *J Am Coll Cardiol* 1991;**18**: 1077–84.

5 Canto JG, Every NR, Magid DJ *et al.* The volume of primary angioplasty procedures and survival after acute myocardial infarction. *N Engl J Med* 2000;**342**: 1573–80.

27 What are the contraindications to thrombolytic therapy for acute myocardial infarction? Is diabetic retinopathy a contraindication?

Kenneth W Mahaffey

Haemorrhagic complications (particularly intracranial) are the most important risks associated with thrombolysis. The 1996 ACC/AHA guidelines for the management of acute myocardial infarction list four absolute contraindications to thrombolytic therapy:

- Previous haemorrhagic stroke or other stroke within one year
- Known intracranial neoplasm
- Active internal bleeding (excluding menses)
- Suspected aortic dissection.

In cases where the nature of the stroke (haemorrhagic or otherwise) is unknown, then the risk of *not* administering a thrombolytic agent should be considered. The majority of strokes are occlusive in origin, and thus lack of certain knowledge should probably not represent a contraindication to thrombolysis in those patients (such as those with extensive territories of myocardial infarction who present early) who have most to gain.

In addition, there are relative contraindications for which the potential risks need to be assessed against the anticipated benefits:

- Uncontrolled hypertension or history of chronic severe hypertension
- Known bleeding diathesis or anticoagulant therapy with INR ≥ 2–3
- Trauma or internal bleeding (within 2–4 weeks), major surgery (<3 weeks), prolonged CPR (>10 minutes), non-compressible vascular puncture, active peptic ulcer
- Pregnancy
- For streptokinase/anistreplase – prior exposure (with 5 days to 2 years) or prior allergic reaction.

Ocular haemorrhage after thrombolysis has been reported, and diabetic retinopathy was once considered a relative contra-indication to thrombolytic therapy in AHA/ACC guidelines.

Although no systematic evaluation has been performed, the GUSTO-I trial observed no intraocular haemorrhages in 6011 patients with diabetes. Currently, therefore, diabetic retinopathy is only considered a contraindication to thrombolysis if there is clear evidence of recent retinal haemorrhage.

Further reading

Fibrinolytic Therapy Trialists' (FTT) Collaborative Group. Indications for fibrinolytic therapy in suspected acute myocardial infarction: collaborative overview of early mortality and major morbidity results from all randomised trials of more than 1000 patients. *Lancet* 1994;**343**: 311–22.

Gunnar RM, Passamani ER, Bourdillon PDV *et al.* Guidelines for the early management of patients with acute myocardial infarction. A report of the American College of Cardiology/American Heart Association task force on assessment of diagnostic and therapeutic cardiovascular procedures. *J Am Coll Cardiol* 1990;**16**: 249–292.

Mahaffey KW, Granger CB, Toth CA *et al.* for the GUSTO-I Investigators. Diabetic retinopathy should not be a contraindication for thrombolytic therapy for acute myocardial infarction: review of ocular hemorrhage incidence and location in the GUSTO-I trial. *J Am Coll Cardiol* 1997;**30**: 1606–10.

Ryan TJ, Anderson JL, Antman EM *et al.* ACC/AHA guidelines for the management of patients with acute myocardial infarction. *J Am Coll Cardiol* 1996;**28**: 1328–1428.

Sane DC, Califf RM, Topol EJ, Stump DC, Mark DB, Greenberg CS. Bleeding during thrombolytic therapy for acute myocardial infarction: mechanisms and management. *Ann Intern Med* 1989;**111**: 1010–22.

28 Exercise testing after myocardial infarction: how soon, what protocol, how should results be acted upon?

Adam D Timmis

Risk stratification in acute myocardial infarction aims to identify patients at greatest risk of recurrent ischaemic events who might benefit prognostically from further investigation and treatment. Risk, however, is not a linear function of time, more than 60% of all major events during the first year occurring in the first 30 days after hospital admission.[1] Recognition of this fact has rendered obsolete old arguments about the appropriate timing of stress testing and other non-invasive tests which must be performed as early as possible (certainly before discharge) to be of significant value. Not all patients need a stress test, which is unlikely to provide significant incremental information when unrelieved chest pain or severe heart failure, for example, confirm a high level of risk.

However, there remains a group that makes a largely un-complicated early recovery for whom pre-discharge stress testing is recommended as a means of detecting residual myocardial ischaemia.[2] A symptom limited test using the Bruce protocol is recommended for most patients although for some, particularly the elderly, modified protocols may be more suitable. An abnormal stress test with regional ST depression may be predictive of recurrent ischaemic events and provides grounds for coronary arteriography with a view to revascularisation. Other markers of risk include low exercise tolerance (<7 mets), failure of the blood pressure to rise normally during exercise and exertional arrhythmias. Unfortunately, recent meta-analysis has shown that inducible ischaemia during treadmill testing has a low positive predictive value for death and myocardial infarction in the first year, falling below 10% in patients who have received thrombolytic therapy.[3] Nevertheless, when "non-ischaemic" risk criteria are considered, the treadmill may provide added clinical value, inability to perform a stress test and low exercise tolerance both being independently predictive of recurrent events.[4] Moreover, the negative predictive accuracy of pre-discharge stress testing is high, those with a normal test usually having a good prognosis without need for additional investigation.[5] Finally, it should be noted that the diagnostic value of exertional ST depression and reversible thallium perfusion defects is equivalent, making the treadmill a more cost effective strategy for risk stratification than the gamma camera.[3]

References

1 Stevenson R, Ranjadayalan K, Wilkinson P *et al*. Short and long term prognosis of acute myocardial infarction since introduction of thrombolysis. *BMJ* 1993;**307**: 349–53.

2 Peterson ED, Shaw LJ, Califf RM. Clinical guideline: part II. Risk stratification after myocardial infarction. *Ann Intern Med* 1997;**126**: 561–82.

3 Shaw LJ, Peterson ED, Kesler K *et al*. A metaanalysis of predischarge risk stratification after acute myocardial infarction with stress electro-cardiographic, myocardial perfusion, and ventricular function imaging. *Am J Cardiol* 1996;**78**: 1327–37.

4 Stevenson R, Wilkinson P, Marchant B *et al*. Relative value of clinical variables, treadmill stress testing and Holter ST monitoring for post-infarction risk stratification. *Am J Cardiol* 1994;**74**: 221–5.

5 Stevenson R, Umachandran V, Ranjadayalan K *et al*. Reassessment of treadmill stress testing for risk stratification in patients with acute myocardial infarction treated by thrombolysis. *Br Heart J* 1993;**70**: 415–20.

29 What are the risks of recurrent ischaemic events after myocardial infarction: prehospital, at 30 days and at 1 year?

Adam D Timmis

Data from the WHO MONICA project in 38 populations from 21 countries show that 49% and 54%, respectively, of all men and women with an acute coronary event die within 28 days.[1] About 70% of these deaths occur out of hospital on day 1 and it is generally accepted that a large proportion of these early deaths are the result of ventricular fibrillation. Thus provision of rapid access to a defibrillator remains the single most effective way to save lives in acute coronary syndromes. Following hospital admission the outcome of acute myocardial infarction is determined largely by left ventricular function. Before the introduction of thrombolytic and other reperfusion strategies, average in-hospital mortality from acute myocardial infarction declined from 32% during the 1960s to 18% during the 1980s.[2] With the introduction of reperfusion therapy further improvements in the short and long term prognosis of acute myocardial infarction have been confirmed in several large studies comparing cohorts of patients admitted before and after the late 1980s.[3,4] Thus, in a group of patients who received CCU treatment for acute myocardial infarction, we reported 30 day and 1 year mortality rates (95% confidence intervals) of 16.0% (13.4–19.2%) and 21.7% (18.6–25.2%), rising to 19.6% (16.6–23.0%) and 33.2% (29.5–37.2%), respectively, when a combined end point of mortality plus non-fatal recurrent events (unstable angina, myocardial infarction) was considered.[5] Multivariate predictors of better short term survival included treatment with thrombolysis and aspirin, while predictors of worse survival included left ventricular failure, advanced age and bundle branch block. Whether survival after acute myocardial infarction has continued to improve in the thrombolytic era is unknown although the increasing application of effective secondary prevention strategies provides grounds for optimism.

References

1 Tunstall-Pedoe H, Kuulasmaa K, Amouyel P *et al.* Myocardial infarctions and coronary deaths in the World Health Organisation MONICA Project. Registration procedures, event rates, and case fatality rates in

38 populations from 21 countries in four continents. *Circulation* 1994;**90**: 583–612.

2 De Vreede JJM, Gorgels APM, Verstraaten GMP *et al.* Did prognosis after acute myocardial infarction change during the past 30 years? A meta-analysis. *J Am Coll Cardiol* 1991;**18**: 698–706.

3 Naylor CD, Chen E. Population-wide mortality trends among patients hospitalized for acute myocardial infarction: the Ontario experience, 1981 to 1991. *J Am Coll Cardiol* 1994;**15**: 1431–8.

4 Rosamond WD, Chambless LE, Folsom AR *et al.* Trends in the incidence of myocardial infarction and in mortality due to coronary heart disease, 1987 to 1994. *N Engl J Med* 1998;**339**: 861–7.

5 Stevenson R, Ranjadayalan K, Wilkinson P *et al.* Short and long term prognosis of acute myocardial infarction since introduction of thrombolysis. *BMJ* 1993;**307**: 349–53.

30 What is appropriate secondary prevention after acute myocardial infarction?

Michael Schachter

At least half the patients who suffer an acute infarct will survive at least one month, though 10–20% will die within the next year. It is to be hoped and expected that more active early intervention will bring about further improvements in short term survival. There is therefore a large and growing number of patients where there is a need to prevent further cardiovascular events and to maintain and improve the quality of life.

Aspirin

Aspirin at low to medium doses (75–325mg daily) reduces mortality, reinfarction and particularly stroke by 10–45% after myocardial infarction. It has been estimated that there is about one serious haemorrhage, gastrointestinal or intracerebral, for every event prevented. At the moment there is no comparable evidence for dipyridamole, ticlopidine or clopidogrel.

Beta blockers

There is overwhelming evidence for the beneficial effect of beta blockers, both within the first few hours of myocardial infarction and for up to three years afterwards. Reduction in mortality ranges from 15 to 45%, almost all of it accounted for by fewer instances of sudden death. All beta blockers appear equally suitable, except those with partial agonist activity. The contraindications are controversial, but most would include asthma, severe heart block and otherwise untreated heart failure, but patients with poor left ventricular function benefit most. In asthmatic patients, particularly, heart rate limiting calcium channel blockers (verapamil or diltiazem) may be useful alternatives to beta blockers in the absence of uncontrolled heart failure.

Lipid-lowering drugs

The large secondary prevention trials with simvastatin and prava-statin (4S, CARE, LIPID) have demonstrated unequivocally the value of cholesterol lowering even in patients with "average" total LDL cholesterol levels of about 5mmol/l. It is arguable that any patient who has had a myocardial infarct should be offered treatment with a statin on the basis that their level of LDL cholesterol is too high for them. However, this is not orthodox practice at present. The previous practice of only measuring cholesterol levels some months after an infarct should be abandoned and the levels assayed *on admission* at the same time as cardiac enzymes. This gives a reliable figure for usual cholesterol levels: a delay of a couple of days in sampling will not. Following the VA-HIT study treating patients with HDL cholesterol levels ≤1 mmol/l with a fibrate should be considered but again is not yet established practice.

ACE inhibitors

These drugs would of course be used in patients with symptomatic heart failure but should also be used in asymptomatic patients with ejection fractions <40%. This is associated with significant decreases in mortality (20–30%) and in sudden death, as well as in reinfarction. All ACE inhibitors so far tested share these effects. Treatment should be started within 1–2 days of the infarct and should be continued indefinitely. Whether all patients should be given these drugs post-infarction, in the absence of contraindications, is a more difficult issue. In unselected populations the benefits of treatment are much less clear cut. However, data from the recent HOPE trial[1] suggest substantial risk reduction for higher risk vascular patients – which may include a large proportion of patients who have suffered a myocardial infarction. Other ongoing trials (such as EUROPA, using Perindopril) may help clarify this issue.

Other action

In addition to these relatively specific measures, diabetes and hypertension must of course be treated as required, and smoking discouraged. Some have advocated the use of fish oils especially in dyslipidaemic patients, either as supplements or as fish. The use of warfarin has been controversial for many years. It is highly effective in preventing cardiovascular events, particularly stroke, but at the cost of more adverse effects than aspirin and the inconvenience of monitoring. It is therefore not recommended for first-line use by most cardiologists.

Finally, it should be remembered that all of this translates into a considerable burden for our patients. Evidence-based medicine will lead to the prescription of 4 or more drugs, usually indefinitely. We must be prepared to make a case for the patient to accept that it really is worthwhile. At the moment, for whatever reasons, most of these proven measures are underused.

References

1 Heart Outcomes Prevention Evaluation Study Investigators. Effects of ramipril on cardiovascular and microvascular outcomes in people with diabetes mellitus: results of the HOPE study and MICRO-HOPE substudy. *Lancet* 2000;**355**: 253–9.

Further reading

Frishman WH, Cheng A. Secondary prevention of myocardial infarction: role of beta-adrenergic blockers and angiotensin converting enzyme inhibitors. *Am Heart J* 1999;**137**: S25–34

Kendall MJ, Horton RC, eds. *Preventing coronary artery disease. Cardioprotective therapeutics in practice.* London: Martin Dunitz, 1998.

Michaels AD. The secondary prevention of myocardial infarction. *Current Probl Cardiol* 1999;**10**: 617–77

Velasco JA. After 4S, CARE and LIPID is evidence-based medicine being practised? *Atherosclerosis* 1999;**147 (suppl 1)**: S39–44

31 What advice should I give patients about driving and flying after myocardial infarction?

John Cockcroft

Compared to other forms of international travel, flying presents fewer demands on the invalid passenger than the alternative modes of travel. Airlines have a duty of care to other passengers who may be inconvenienced by emergency diversions, unscheduled stops and delays in the event of a medical emergency.

Recertification of drivers and pilots following myocardial infarction depends upon their subsequent risk of incapacitation whilst at the controls. All pilots and all professional drivers have a duty to inform the relevant licencing authority as soon as possible following myocardial infarction.

There are no international regulations governing the prospective passenger who has recently suffered a myocardial infarction and no statutory duty to inform the airline concerned. Most will be guided in the decision whether to fly or not by their cardiologist or family doctor. Modern passenger aircraft have a cabin atmospheric pressure equivalent to 5–8,000 feet, and alveolar oxygen tension falls by around 30%. This may exacerbate symptoms in any patient who experiences angina or shortness of breath whilst walking 50 metres or climbing 10 stairs. The enforced immobility of the passenger on a long flight, airport transfers and the crossing of time zones should be considered.

If fewer than 10 days have elapsed since myocardial infarction, or if there is significant cardiac failure, angina or arrhythmia the patient may require oxygen or suitable accompaniment. The airline should be informed, and will request a report on a standard medical information form (MEDIF).

Professional pilots are disqualified from flying for nine months after myocardial infarction, but may subsequently be allowed to fly in a multi-pilot aircraft provided that investigations, carried out by a cardiologist acceptable to the licencing authority, are satisfactory, as follows:

- Exercise ECG to Bruce protocol stage 4 reveals no evidence of ischaemia
- 24 hr ECG reveals no abnormality

- Echocardiogram shows ejection fraction greater than or equal to 50% and normal wall motion
- Coronary angiography reveals no stenosis greater than 30% in any vessel distant from the infarction
- Any underlying risk factors must have been appropriately treated, and certification will be subject to annual cardiology review, with further coronary angiography within 5 years.

Private pilots are subject to the same regulations but may fly with a suitably qualified safety pilot in a dual control aircraft without undergoing angiography. Symptomatic or treated angina, arrhythmia or cardiac failure disqualifies any pilot from flying.

Professional drivers may be relicenced 3 months after myocardial infarction provided that there is no angina, peripheral vascular disease or heart failure. Arrhythmia, if present, must not have caused symptoms within the last 2 years. Treatment is allowed provided that it causes no symptoms likely to impair performance.

- Exercise ECG to Bruce protocol stage 3 must reveal no symptoms or signs of ischaemia.
- Recertification will be subject to periodic satisfactory medical reports.

Private drivers need not inform the licencing authority after myocardial infarction, but should not drive for one month. If arrhythmia causes symptoms likely to affect performance, or if angina occurs whilst driving, the licencing authority must be informed, and driving must cease until symptoms are adequately controlled.

Further reading
Joint Aviation Authorities. Joint Aviation Requirements FCL3(Medical) 1997.
The Medical Commission on Accident Prevention. Medical aspects of fitness to drive 1995.

32 What is the mortality rate for cardiogenic shock complicating myocardial infarction? How should such patients be managed to improve outcome and what are the results?

Prithwish Banerjee and Michael S Norrell

The advent of the thrombolytic era has not altered the incidence or mortality rate for cardiogenic shock complicating myocardial infarction (MI). It still represents almost 10% of patients with MI, with almost 90% dying within 30 days. [1]

Pooled results from retrospective, unrandomised data or historical reviews, which examined the effects of early re-vascularisation, have suggested reduced mortality following bypass surgery (CABG) or coronary angioplasty (PTCA) to 33%[2] and 42% [3] respectively. Recently, a few randomised trials have attempted to compare such early (within 48 hours) revascularisation with a strategy of initial medical stabilisation. The latter might include thrombolysis, inotropic support and intra-aortic balloon pump counterpulsation (IABP), still with the option of delayed inter-vention. It is unfortunate that most of these studies have faltered on slow patient recruitment [4] leaving only one completed study (SHOCK, SHould we emergently revascularise Occluded Coronaries for Shock) to guide our management of these patients.[5]

Over a 5 year period, the SHOCK trial randomised 302 patients to receive either early revascularisation within hours from randomisation, or initial medical stabilisation with the option of delayed intervention. Thirty day mortality was reduced in the early intervention group (46% vs 56%) with this benefit extending out to 6 months and particularly apparent in the younger (<75 years) age group. The low mortality in the control group is striking, and explains the lack of a large difference between the two groups. Nevertheless, it suggests benefit even with a relatively aggressive conservative policy in these patients.

Because of trial recruitment difficulties it is unlikely that further randomised data will emerge in the foreseeable future. Evidence from the SHOCK trial would seem to suggest that at present it would be reasonable to consider an aggressive approach with early revascularisation in patients with shock complicating myocardial infarction. However, access to surgery should be available – 36% of patients required this intervention rather than PTCA. Mean time to revascularisation was under 1 hour in the trial, and quite how much later such benefit might extend is unclear. Care should include vigorous medical stabilisation in all such patients with thrombolysis, inotropes, balloon pumping and even ventilation if necessary with a view to late revascularisation (PTCA or CABG). In young patients early (<48 hours) revascularisation should be considered.

References

1 Walters MI, Burn S, Houghton T *et al*. Cardiogenic shock: are HEROICS justified? *Circulation* 1997;**96(suppl I):** 168A.
2 O'Neil WW. Angioplasty therapy for cardiogenic shock: are randomised trials necessary? *J Am Coll Cardiol* 1992;**19:** 915–17.
3 Bolooki H. Emergency cardiac procedures in patients in cardiogenic shock due to complications of coronary artery disease. *Circulation* 1989;**79(suppl I):** I137–48.
4 Norell MS. Randomised trials in cardiogenic shock: what's the problem? *Eur Heart J* 1999;**20:** 987–8.
5 Hochman J, Boland J, Sleeper L *et al*. Early revascularisation in acute myocardial infarction complicated by cardiogenic shock. *N Engl J Med* 1999;**341:** 625–34.

33 What is the risk of a patient dying or having a myocardial infarction around the time of surgery for coronary artery disease and for valve replacement?

Tom Treasure

General approach to quoting numbers

First some general comments. The figures given should ideally be those currently being achieved by the team to whom the patient is referred. In general terms, registry data are more representative than published series, which inevitably include bias towards more successful figures. The data should be adjusted up or down to match the circumstances of the individual patient, who is helped towards a rational decision based on the anticipated risks and benefits.

What is the risk of death with CABG

The UK Cardiac Surgery Register for the three years up to 1997 gives a 3% mortality for isolated coronary artery surgery, which is applicable to the current case mix. It therefore applies to the typical patients – male, elective, aged 60–70, with an adequate left ventricle. Patients with one or more risk factors for perioperative death, which are older age, female sex, obesity, worse ventricular function, diabetes, very unstable or emergency status, or significant co-morbidity of any type, should have the stated risk appropriately increased.

What is the risk of death with valve replacement?

The United Kingdom Heart Valve Registry provides very reliable thirty day mortality figures which for the three years 1994–1996 inclusive were 5% for aortic valve replacement and 6% for mitral valve replacement.

What is the risk of stroke?

Lethal brain damage and permanently disabling hemiplegia are rare with a combined risk of about 0.5% in current practice. If every focal deficit discovered on brain imaging, or every transient neurological sign is included the incidence would probably be nearer 5%. Most of these focal deficits are caused by atheroembolism. Air, left atrial thrombus and calcific valve debris are additional risk in valve surgery. I quote the routine patient a risk of stroke of 1% to 2% adjusted upwards for increasing age, history of previous stroke or TIA, and hypertension, and adjusted down for relative youth.

The incidence of subtle diffuse or global brain injury depends on definition. Some difficulty with concentration and memory affects about a quarter of patients – but very few are troubled by it to any extent.[1]

What is the risk of myocardial infarction?

This is extremely difficult to define. In good hands it rarely complicates valve operations without coronary artery disease. In coronary surgery incidence depends on definition but myocardial dysfunction, local or global, is the commonest cause of death. The incidence of infarction is entirely dependant on definition and any figure from 2% to 10% could be given, depending on the criteria used.

Reference
1 Treasure T. Cerebral protection in adults. In: Yacoub M, Pepper J, eds. *Annual of cardiac surgery*, 7th edition. London and Philadelphia: Current Science, 1994: 161–9

34 Which patients with post-infarct septal rupture should be treated surgically, and what are the success rates?

Tom Treasure

Myocardial rupture is a more common cause of death after infarction than is generally appreciated.[1] It complicates about 3% of all myocardial infarctions and is the cause of death in about 17% of fatal infarcts. Myocardial rupture can involve the LV wall, the septum and the papillary muscles and occurs in proportion to the amount of muscle at risk with a ratio of about 10:2:1. Rupture of the LV wall is almost always immediately fatal and is the cause of death in about 13% (75% of 17%) of all fatal infarcts, as "electromechanical dissociation".

The minority who rupture only through the septum (loosely known as post-infarct VSD) may be saved by surgery. The hospital mortality for surgical repair is probably 40% (without reporting bias – but there is surgical selection and natural selection – most have had to survive transfer to a surgical centre). The mortality is close to 100% without surgery. Favourable features are younger age, anterior rather than inferior infarcts, more surviving left and right ventricular myocardium, and functioning kidneys. There was a vogue for holding these patients on a balloon pump to operate on them when the infarcted tissue is better able to take stitches. It is a long wait before there is any material advantage, and any benefit in reported figures of percentage operative survival was due to loss of patients along the way. If you are going to operate on these cases, it is probably a case of the sooner the better.

Current data would suggest that concomitant coronary artery bypass grafting does little to improve mortality rates from surgical post-infarct VSD.[2]

Reference
1 Dellborg M, Held P, Swedberg K *et al.* Rupture of the myocardium. Occurrence and risk factors. *Br Heart J* 1985;**54**: 11–16.
2 Dalrymple-Hay MJ, Langley SM, Sami SA *et al.* Should coronary artery bypass grafting be performed at the same time as repair of a post-infarct ventricular septal defect? *Eur J Cardio-Thorac Surg* 1998;**13**: 286–92.

35 What patterns of coronary disease are associated with improved short and long term survival after CABG compared with medical therapy?

Martin Paul Hayward

Many factors have influenced the short and long term results of bypass surgery, not least the improvements in surgical techniques and experience, changes in the population of patients undergoing surgery, many of whom would never have been deemed suitable for surgery even 10 years ago, improvements in postoperative medical management and the use of the left internal mammary artery (LIMA) as the graft of choice for the left anterior descending coronary artery (LAD) in virtually all patients today.

30 day operative mortality

Short term survival after bypass surgery is 1–3% at most institutions around the world. The Society of Thoracic Surgeons National Database mortality figures[1] for 80,881 patients undergoing isolated bypass surgery between 1980 and 1990 were 4.75% for left main disease, 3.32% for triple vessel disease and 2.86% for one and two vessel disease. In-hospital mortality was 2.9% for first time operation and 7.14% for re-operation. Recognised factors affecting in-hospital mortality include older age, female sex, co-morbid renal and cardiovascular disease, diabetes, cardiogenic shock, emergency, salvage or redo operation, preoperative intra-aortic balloon pump use and associated valve disease.

Long term survival after surgery

The late results of bypass surgery depend on the extent of cardiac disease, the effectiveness of the original operation, progression rate of atherosclerosis and the impact of non-cardiac disease. Patient-related variables associated with poorer late survival include reduced ventricular function, congestive cardiac failure, triple vessel or left main stem disease, severity of symptoms, advanced age and diabetes.

The patients who gain most from surgery are those most at risk from dying with medical therapy alone. Pertinent high-risk characteristics included left main stem (LMS) disease, triple vessel disease or double vessel disease that included a proximal LAD lesion, and triple vessel disease associated with impaired LV function. The VA study at 18 years[2] demonstrated superior surgical survival throughout the 18 years, but was only significant overall at 7 years (med. vs surg. survival 53% vs 79% p = 0.007); benefit was much greater in the high risk group with LMS stenosis >50%, single or double vessel disease with impaired LV function, and triple vessel disease with LV EF <40%. In 1988 ECSS[3] reported 12 year results demonstrating significantly higher cumulative survival in the surgical group, notably again in patients with 3 vessel disease (med. vs surg. survival 82% vs 94% (p = 0.0002) at 5 years and 68% vs 78% (p = 0.01) at 10 years). Proximal LAD disease >95% in two or three vessel disease was an outstanding anatomical predictor of survival (med. vs surg. survival at 10 years 65% vs 77% (p = 0.007)), again with significant crossover into the surgery group. The CASS study[4] demonstrated no difference in survival for any subset at 5 years, but did not include any patients with poor LV function, LMS disease, angina greater than class 2, co-morbid disease or unstable angina. It is therefore difficult to extrapolate data from this trial to modern patient populations.

Combining results from seven of these early randomised trials led to the publication of survival figures for 5, 7 and 10 years.[5] Medical vs surgical mortality for all patients was 15.8% vs 10.2% (p = 0.0001) at 5 years, with attenuation of this benefit to a mortality of 30.5% (med.) and 26.4% (surg.) (p = 0.03) at 10 years. Extension of life for all patients having surgery was 4.3 months at 10 years. High-risk patients once again benefited the most from surgery, but in lower risk groups, a survival extension for those with proximal LAD disease (14 months), triple vessel disease (7 months) or LMS disease (19 months) was identified. This survival benefit was independent of degree of LV impairment or abnormal stress testing. Median survival for patients with LMS disease was 13.1 years in the surgical group and 6.2 years for those treated medically. The superior patency of the LIMA graft compared with saphenous vein grafts has been established beyond any doubt and additional survival benefit, up to 18 years, has been demonstrated.[6]

References

1 Edwards FH, Clark RE, Schwarz M. Coronary artery bypass grafting: Society of Thoracic Surgeons National Database experience. *Ann Thorac Surg* 1994;**57**;12–19.

2 The Veterans Administration Coronary Artery Bypass Surgery Cooperative Study Group. Eighteen year follow up in the Veterans Affairs Cooperative study of coronary artery bypass surgery for unstable angina. *Circulation* 1992;**86**: 121–6.

3 The European Coronary Surgery Study Group. Twelve year follow up of survival in the Randomised European Coronary Surgery Study. *N Engl J Med* 1988;**319**: 332–7.

4 CASS principle investigators. Myocardial infarction and mortality in the Coronary Artery Study (CASS) randomised trial. *N Engl J Med* 1984;**310**: 750–8.

5 Yusuf S, Peduzzi P, Fisher LD *et al.* Effect of CABG surgery on survival: overview of 10 year results from randomised trials by the CABG surgery triallists collaborations. *Lancet* 1994;**344**: 563–70.

6 Boylan MJ, Lytle BW, Loop FD *et al.* Surgical treatment of isolated left anterior descending coronary stenosis – comparison of LIMA and venous autografts at 18–20 years follow up. *J Thorac Cardiovasc Surg* 1994;**107**: 657–62.

36 Coronary artery bypass grafting: what is the case for total arterial revascularisation?

DP Taggart

The clinical and prognostic benefits of coronary artery bypass grafting (CABG) for certain subgroups of patients with ischaemic heart disease are well established.[1] Most patients have three vessel coronary artery disease and the conventional CABG operation uses a single internal mammary artery (IMA) and two vein grafts to perform three bypass grafts. This procedure provides excellent short and intermediate term outcome but is limited, in the long term, by vein graft failure. Ten years after CABG 95% of IMA grafts are patent and disease free whereas three quarters of vein grafts are severely diseased or blocked.[2]

The case for one arterial graft

For over a decade the superior patency of a single IMA over vein grafts has been known to improve survival and to reduce the incidence of late myocardial infarction, recurrent angina and the need for further cardiac interventions.[1,2]

The case for two arterial grafts

Substantial evidence for the prognostic and clinical benefits of both IMA grafts has recently been reported in a large study from the Cleveland clinic.[3] In comparison to the use of a single IMA graft, use of both IMA grafts resulted in a further significant improvement in survival (with a reduction in mortality by 10% at 10 years) and a fourfold reduction in the need for reoperation. Furthermore, these benefits extended across all groups of patients with a five year life expectancy including "elderly" patients (up to mid-seventies), and those with diabetes and impaired ventricular function. The major concern of harvesting both IMA is an increase in sternal wound complications. This can be avoided by a skeletonisation rather than a pedicled technique which leaves collateral vessels intact on the sternum and allows the safe use of both IMAs even in diabetic patients.

The case for three arterial grafts

Several arteries have been proposed as the third arterial graft and the most widely used is the radial artery. The radial artery is a versatile conduit, which can be harvested easily and safely, has handling characteristics superior to those of other arterial grafts and comfortably reaches any coronary target. For the patient it offers the prospect of superior graft patency compared to saphenous vein grafts[4] as well as improved wound healing. The potential impact of the radial artery on survival is not yet established as it has only been in widespread use for five years.

Finally, many patients are interested to know "how long grafts are likely to last". This may be viewed most helpfully in terms of event rates, rather than physical lack of occlusion of a graft: "ischaemic event rate" (5% per year) and cardiac mortality (2–2.5% per year). A recurrent "event" (death, MI or recurrence of angina) occurs in 25% of surgically treated patients in <5 years, and 50% at 10 years.

In summary, the use of arterial grafts offers substantial short and long term clinical and prognostic benefits. In particular the use of both IMA grafts significantly reduces mortality and the need for re-operation. Current evidence suggests that the superior patency of arterial grafts also reduces perioperative mortality by reducing perioperative myocardial infarction. This is particularly true in patients with smaller or more severely diseased coronary arteries (females, diabetics, Asian background) where discrepancy between the size of vein grafts and coronary vessels leads to "run-off" problems and a predisposition to graft thrombosis. Careful harvesting of both IMAs can be performed even in diabetic patients without an increase in wound healing problems. Relative contraindications to arterial grafts are patients who are likely to require significant inotropic support in the postoperative period (because of the risk of graft vasoconstriction) or those with severely impaired ventricular function (ejection fraction less than 25%) and limited life expectancy.

References

1 Yusuf S, Zucker D, Peduzzi P *et al.* Effect of coronary artery bypass graft surgery on survival: overview of 10-year results from randomised trials by the Coronary Artery Bypass Graft Surgery Trialists Collaboration. *Lancet* 1994;**344**: 563–70.
2 Nwasokwa ON. Coronary artery bypass graft disease. *Ann Intern Med* 1995;**123**: 528–45.

3 Lytle BW, Blackstone EH, Loop FD *et al.* Two internal thoracic artery grafts are better than one. *J Thorac Cardiovasc Surg* 1999;**117**: 855–72.
4 Taggart DP. The radial artery as a conduit for coronary artery bypass grafting. *Heart* 1999;**82**: 409–10.

37 How common are neuropsychological complications after cardiopulmonary bypass (CPB)? How predictable and severe are they? Can they be prevented?

Stan Newman and Jan Stygall

Neuropsychological complications have been found to occur in a proportion of patients following CPB. These problems reveal themselves as impaired cognitive function, i.e. difficulties with memory, attention, concentration, and speed of motor and mental response. However, the reported frequency with which these problems occur varies considerably. Studies assessing patients 5–10 days postoperatively have suggested an incidence of neuropsychological deficits ranging from 12.5 to 90%. Later assessments, at about 2 to 6 months after surgery, have indicated deficits in 12 to 37% of patients studied.

How predictable are they?

The variation in reported incidence has been ascribed to several factors such as number, type, sensitivity, and timing of neuro-psychological tests used, as well as the definition of neuro-psychological deficit and the method of statistical analysis employed. These methodological issues have been addressed at international consensus conferences in 1994 and 1997. Patient related variables such as age and disease severity have also been associated with cognitive decline post-cardiac surgery. Therefore centres employing different criteria for surgery may report differing rates of deficit.

Deficits detected within a few days of surgery are also problematic in that they are often transient in nature. These assessments appear to be contaminated by postoperative readjustment and anaesthetic residue as well as genuine neuropsychological difficulties. Long term deficits (over 6 weeks) are considered to be more stable and to reflect a more persistent neuropsychological problem.

How severe are they?

Given that these problems reflect a decline in performance of approximately 20–25% from that prior to surgery, they can be considered severe. What is more difficult is how they translate into the patient's everyday life. This is dependent upon the nature of their activities. A cardiac surgeon who suffered a 20% decline in their fine motor movements would undoubtedly have a severe disability. In contrast a road sweeper would not suffer unduly, at least in their work. The tests customarily performed in this area are most useful as a window onto surgery rather than showing an impact on quality of life.

Can they be prevented?

The mechanisms for neuropsychological decline are considered to be multifactorial. The most popular explanation for cognitive dysfunction is microemboli delivered to the brain during surgery. These can be either air or particulate (atheromatous matter, fat, platelet aggregates, etc.) in nature. In an attempt to reduce the incidence of neuropsychological decline various interventional studies have been designed. Much of this work has centred on the impact of different equipment and techniques used in surgery on neuropsychological outcome. Early studies comparing bubble and membrane oxygenators indicated a higher frequency of microemboli detected when using bubble oxygenators with decreased neuropsychological deficits occurring in the membrane group. Studies have also found that the introduction of an arterial line filter into the CPB circuit significantly reduces the number of microemboli detected at the middle cerebral artery during CABG. A significant reduction in neuropsychological deficits in the filter group has also been reported. In contrast a study comparing pulsatile and non-pulsatile flow found no difference in neuropsychological outcome between the two techniques.

As the use of hypothermic perfusion during CPB has been based on the protective effects of low temperature in limiting the effects of cerebral ischaemia it is surprising that studies so far have failed to find any advantage for hypothermic bypass on neuropsychological outcome. Two studies have examined the impact of pH management on cognitive performance and both have reported benefit from using the alpha stat technique. Less disruption to autoregulation has also been reported in the alpha stat group.

More recently pharmacological neuroprotection has been attempted in these patients with a variety of compounds. Most of these studies have been underpowered and only one appears to have produced some suggestion of neuroprotection.

Further reading
Arrowsmith JE, Harrison MJG, Newman SP *et al*. Neuroprotection of the brain during cardiopulmonary bypass. A randomized trial of Remacemide during coronary artery bypass in 171 patients. *Stroke* 1998;**29**: 2357–62.
Murkin JM, Newman SP, Stump DA *et al*. Statement of consensus on assessment of neurobehavioral outcomes after cardiac surgery. *Ann Thorac Surg* 1995;**59**: 1289–95.
Murkin JM, Stump DA, Blumenthal JA *et al*. Defining dysfunction: group means versus incidence analysis: a statement of consensus. *Ann Thorac Surg* 1997;**64**: 904–5.
Newman SP, Harrison MJG, eds. *The brain and cardiac surgery*. London; Harwood Academic, 2000.

38 Are there benefits to switching from sulphonylureas to insulin after coronary artery bypass grafting?

Jonathan Unsworth-White

Sulphonylureas help to control blood glucose levels by binding to adenosine-5-triphosphate(ATP)-sensitive potassium channels (K_{ATP}-channels) in the beta-cells of the pancreas. This inhibits potassium flux across the cell membrane, leading to depolarisation of the plasmalemma and subsequently the release of endogenous insulin. These same K_{ATP}-channels are also found in the myocardium and in vascular smooth muscle cells and are therefore implicated in the regulation of the cardiovascular system.

A fall in myocardial cytosolic levels of ATP and a rise in extracellular adenosine opens the K_{ATP}-channels during myocardial ischaemia. This is thought to be a natural protective action, related to the phenomena of preconditioning and hibernation. Glibenclamide abolishes this effect at clinically relevant doses and infarct size is increased in animal models of myocardial ischaemia. These drugs also antagonise the vasodilating effects of drugs like minoxidil and diazoxide and can reduce resting myocardial blood flow. In contrast, sulphonylureas might reduce the incidence of post-ischaemic ventricular arrhythmias. By blocking K_{ATP}-channels, they prevent the tendency towards shortening of the action potential during myocardial ischaemia secondary to potassium efflux through opened channels.

Secondly, since type II diabetics are both insulin deficient and insulin resistant, glycaemic control may be improved in some individuals by combining oral medication with insulin or by switching completely.

In summary there remain theoretical arguments for and against changing from sulphonylureas following coronary surgery. The position may be eased by the development of more pancreas-specific drugs. For the time being at least, strict glycaemic control by whatever means should remain the primary aim, if necessary using short acting, low dose sulphonylurea derivatives.

Further reading
Brady PA, Terzic A. The sulphonylurea controversy: more questions from the heart. *J Am Coll Cardiol* 1998;**31**: 950–6.
Smits P, Thien T. Cardiovascular effects of sulphonylurea derivatives. Implications for the treatment of NIDDM? *Diabetologia* 1995;**38**: 116–21.

39 How does recent myocardial infarction affect the perioperative risks of coronary artery bypass grafting?

Jonathan Unsworth-White

Common sense suggests that the more recent the infarction, the higher the operative risk. This is because the infarcted area is surrounded by a critically ischaemic zone. The ultimate survival of this zone depends on many factors, not least of which is the global function of the remaining myocardium. This function is temporarily further compromised by the process of cardio-pulmonary bypass for coronary artery surgery. The likely outcome during this critical phase, therefore, is extension of the infarcted area, with obvious implications for survival of the patient.

It is the duration of this critical phase which is most in doubt. In a recent small retrospective analysis, Herlitz *et al*[1] found that amongst patients with a history of myocardial infarction, infarction within 30 days of surgery was not an independent predictor of total mortality within 2 years of surgery. However, Braxton *et al*[2] made a distinction between Q wave and non-Q wave infarctions in the perioperative period. Although both types rendered the use of balloon pumps and inotropes to wean from bypass more likely, only Q wave infarctions were associated with significantly increased surgical mortality and even then only if surgery was performed within 48 hours of the infarction.

An older but much larger series from Floten *et al*[3] seems to support a high risk for the initial 24–48 hours or so, but more importantly emphasises the relationship between the number of diseased vessels and the risk of surgery after recent infarction. Applebaum *et al*[4] found ejection fraction less than 30%, cardiogenic shock and age greater than 70 years to be significant determinants of death in patients operated upon within 30 days of infarction. These are not surprising factors, fitting as they do with the concept that it is the extent of the jeopardised myocardium which is the determinant of risk, especially within the first day or two after the myocardial infarction.

References

1 Herlitz J, Brandrup G, Haglid M *et al.* Death, mode of death, morbidity, and rehospitalization after coronary artery bypass grafting in relation

to occurrence of and time since a previous myocardial infarction. *J Thorac Cardiovasc Surg* 1997;**45**: 109–13.

2 Braxton JH, Hammond GL, Franco KL *et al*. Optimal timing of coronary artery bypass graft surgery after acute myocardial infarction. *Circulation* 1995;**92**: II66-II68.

3 Floten HS, Ahmad A, Swanson JS *et al*. Long-term survival after postinfarction bypass operation: early versus late operation. *Ann Thorac Surg* 1989;**48**: 757–62.

4 Applebaum R, House R, Rademaker A *et al*. Coronary artery bypass grafting within 30 days of acute myocardial infarction. Early and late results in 406 patients. *J Thorac and Cardiovasc Surg* 1991;**102**: 745–52.

40 How soon before cardiac surgery should aspirin be stopped?

Jonathan Unsworth-White

Aspirin irreversibly inhibits platelet function by blocking the cyclooxygenase pathway. It is a vital adjunct in the prevention of coronary thrombosis[1] and is known to reduce the risk of acute bypass graft closure.[2] Unfortunately it also causes increased bleeding after cardiac surgery and increases the risk of emergency re-sternotomy in the first few hours.[3] For this reason many centres try to stop aspirin for a few days prior to surgery.

Platelets have a life span in the plasma of approximately 10 days. Therefore if aspirin were discontinued 10 days prior to surgery, the affected platelet pool would be completely replenished with fresh platelets by the time of the operation. This however leaves the patient vulnerable to an acute myocardial event during the latter part of this time and may also make graft occlusion more likely in the immediate postoperative period. It also supposes that operating lists can be planned 10 days in advance.

In reality, patients are usually asked to stop aspirin 5–7 days in advance. This seems to be a suitable compromise for the majority of patients although for a few (tight left main stem stenosis or past history of TIAs or stroke), the risk of stopping aspirin may outweigh the potential benefits.

References

1 Antiplatelet Trialists' Collaboration. Collaborative overview of randomised trials of antiplatelet therapy-1: Prevention of death, myocardial infarction, and stroke by prolonged antiplatelet therapy in various categories of patients. *BMJ* 1994;**308**: 81–106.

2 Antiplatelet Trialists' Collaboration. Collaborative overview of randomised trials of antiplatelet therapy-II: Maintenance of vascular graft or arterial patency by antiplatelet therapy. *BMJ* 1994;**308**: 159–68.

3 Kallis P, Tooze JA, Talbot S, *et al.* Pre-operative aspirin decreases platelet aggregation and increases post-operative blood loss – a prospective, randomised, placebo controlled, double-blind clinical trial in 100 patients with chronic stable angina. *Eur J Cardio-thoracic Surg* 1994;**8**: 404–9.

41 When should we operate to relieve mitral regurgitation?

Tom Treasure

There are three circumstances when surgery is required for mitral regurgitation:

1 To save life in the acute case

Sudden mitral regurgitation following rupture of degenerative chordae tendineae, papillary muscle rupture, or endocarditis may be very poorly tolerated. The surgeon may be presented with a patient in pulmonary oedema, even ventilated, and then an operation may be the only way to save life.

2 The symptomatic patient with chronic mitral regurgitation

Surgical relief of regurgitant valve lesions can bring dramatic relief. The decision is not always easy but a sensible appraisal of the risks and benefits is what is needed. If there is a tolerably good ventricle, and substantial regurgitation to correct, then the benefits are likely to outweigh the risks. The degree of left venticular dilatation to be tolerated before surgery is required has reduced. In general, it is now suggested that a left ventricular end-systolic dimension (LVESD) of 4.5cm is a sensible threshold for "perhaps not waiting any longer".

3 Mitral regurgitation and the dilated ventricle

The third scenario is the most difficult. Some patients seem to tolerate mitral regurgitation quite well with a large ventricle ejecting partly into a large, relatively low pressure left atrium. The left ventricle may not be as good as it appears because the high ejection fraction is into low afterload. If you continue to wait the risks only get higher. Any increasing tendency in LVESD is ominous and the onset or progression of symptoms should prompt operation to protect the future.

Further reading

Schlant RC. Timing of surgery for nonischemic severe mitral regurgitation. *Circulation* 1999;**99**: 338–9.

Treasure T. Timing of surgery in chronic mitral regurgitation: In: Wells FC, Shapiro LM. *Mitral valve disease.* Oxford: Butterworth Heinemann, 1996: 187–200.

Tribouilloy CM, Enriquez-Sarano M, Schaff HV *et al.* Impact of preoperative symptoms on survival after surgical correction of mitral regurgitation. *Circulation* 1999;**99**: 400–5.

42 When to repair the mitral valve?

Robin Kanagasabay

Mitral valve repair has been popularised by Carpentier and others and now represents a recognised option in the treatment of mitral valve disease. Advocates argue that all mitral valves should be considered for repair first, and only those that are not suitable should be replaced. Mitral valve repair offers real advantages over replacement, chiefly low operative risk (around 2%[1,2]), avoidance of the risks of long term anticoagulation (in patients who are in sinus rhythm), very low risk of endocarditis, and probably better long term preservation of left ventricular function. The last aspect may not be as clear cut as once thought as techniques to replace the mitral valve while still preserving the sub-valvular chordal apparatus, which is so important in regulating ventricular geometry, may offer many of the advantages once held to be the sole preserve of repair techniques.[3] A potential disadvantage of mitral valve repair is the less certain surgical outcome of the technique which relies on a greater degree of judgement, and the possible need for future redo surgery in around 10% of cases.[4] The standard use of annuloplasty rings has improved results and reduced the need for redo surgery, but not to zero, and this point needs to be discussed with patients prior to choosing an approach.

Different valvular lesions are more or less amenable to mitral valve repair, and require that different techniques be employed:[5]

Increased leaflet motion (Carpentier type II)

The patient with pure mitral regurgitation due to either a floppy myxomatous valve, or posterior leaflet chordal rupture represents the easiest and most successful case and the valve can be repaired by quadrangular resection of the posterior leaflet. Repair of anterior leaflet prolapse is a more complex undertaking and requires either a transfer of chordae from the posterior to the anterior leaflet, or the use of synthetic chordae. An alternative is to suture the free edges of the two leaflets together at their mid-points creating a double orifice valve, the so called Alfieri bow-tie repair.

Normal leaflet motion (Carpentier type I)

In some patients annular dilatation contributes to mitral regurgitation and requires correction with an annuloplasty ring.

Decreased leaflet motion (Carpentier type III)

This is the most difficult lesion to correct. It may require a combination of leaflet augmentation using patches of pericardium, and also elongation or replacement of any restricted chordae. Restricted leaflet motion due to poor ventricular function remains a particularly difficult problem to correct by repair techniques.

Features which indicate a low chance of successful repair

These include:

- Rheumatic valvular disease
- Thickened valve leaflets
- Multiple mechanisms of valve dysfunction
- Extensive prolapse of both leaflets
- Commissural regurgitation
- Annular calcification
- Dissection of valve leaflets complicating endocarditis.

In general all valves that can be repaired should be, although some patients may opt for valve replacement to avoid the (small) risk of needing further surgery due to failure of the repair. Because of the low operative risk, absence of the need for anticoagulation and avoidance of the risks of prosthetic valve endocarditis following valve repair, a further group of patients may be offered valve repair at an early stage of their disease where, on the balance of risks, valve replacement would not yet be justified.

References

1 David TE, Omran A, Armstrong S *et al.* Long-term results of mitral valve repair for myxomatous disease with and without chordal replacement with expanded polytetrafluoroethylene sutures. *J Thorac Cardiovasc Surg* 1998;**115**: 1279–85; discussion 1285–6.
2 Chitwood WR Jr. Mitral valve repair: an odyssey to save the valves! *J Heart Valve Dis* 1998;**7**: 255–61.

3 Lee EM, Shapiro LM, Wells FC. Superiority of mitral valve repair in surgery for degenerative mitral regurgitation. *Eur Heart J* 1997;**18**: 655–63.
4 Gillinov AM, Cosgrove DM, Lytle BW *et al*. Reoperation for failure of mitral valve repair. *J Thorac Cardiovasc Surg* 1997;**113**: 467–73; discussion 473–5.
5 Barlow CW, Imber CJ, Sharples LD *et al*. Cost implications of mitral valve replacement versus repair in mitral regurgitation. *Circulation* 1997;**96(9 suppl)**: II90–3; discussion II94–5.

43 What is the Ross procedure? When is it indicated and what are the advantages?

R Cesnjevar and Victor T Tsang

What is the Ross procedure?

The Ross procedure, or pulmonary autograft procedure, was introduced by Mr Donald Ross in 1967. The operation is performed via median sternotomy on cardiopulmonary bypass. The principle is to replace the diseased aortic valve with the autologous pulmonary valve. The pulmonary autograft is placed in the aortic position as a root replacement with interrupted sutures and the coronary arteries are reimplanted. Great care must be taken during harvesting of the pulmonary root because of the close proximity of the first septal branch of the left anterior descending coronary artery. A homograft (preferably pulmonary) is used to restore continuity between the right ventricular outflow tract and the pulmonary artery. The overall operative risk cited in the current literature is 1.5–7.0%, depending on the patient's age and surgical indication.

In whom should I consider it?

The Ross procedure is the preferred option for aortic valve replacement in the growing child due to the growth potential of the implanted autograft. It should also be considered in any patient where anticoagulation is completely or relatively contraindicated. Another possible indication is active endocarditis because of its "curative" potential. The likelihood of recurrence of endocarditis and of perivalvar leak is lower in patients after a Ross procedure, compared to mechanical valve replacement.

What are the advantages?

The haemodynamic performance of the autograft valve is superior to mechanical valves, with much lower transvalvar gradients and better regression in ventricular size and hypertrophy in the mid-term. Anticoagulation with warfarin (a major contributor to mechanical valve-related morbidity and mortality) is not required after the Ross procedure. More than 90% of all patients are free of any complications (death, degeneration, valve failure, endocarditis) after ten years. However, the subpulmonary homograft may need replacement in the future. The Ross procedure is technically demanding. It is the method of choice for aortic valve replacement in the young, with excellent early postoperative haemodynamic results and good mid-term results. Long term results of the Ross procedure using current techniques are awaited.

Further reading
Elkins RC. The Ross operation: a twelve year experience. *Ann Thorac Surg* 1999;**68(suppl 3)**: S14–18.
Ross DN. Replacement of aortic and mitral valve with a pulmonary autograft. *Lancet* 1967;**ii**: 956–8.

44 What is the risk of stroke each year after a) tissue or b) mechanical MVR or AVR? What is the annual risk of bacterial endocarditis on these prosthetic valves?

Tom Treasure

The risk of stroke after valve replacement is higher in mechanical than tissue valves (in spite of best efforts at anticoagulation) and is higher after mitral than aortic valve replacement. The risk is very much higher in the first year.

To some extent these numbers depend on definition and how hard you look. I quote from our own prospective randomised trial **(in press)** of St Jude and Starr-Edwards valves so the information was deliberately sought and the follow up was very near complete. The annual incident rate of complications (per 100 patient years) is shown in Table 45.1.

Table 44.1   The annual incident rate of complications (per 100 patient years)

	Stroke	TIA	N	"Events"
Mechanical mitral	2.4	4.2	380	6.5
Mechanical aortic	1.0	1.3	870	2.0
Tissue mitral	0	2.5	600	2.5
Tissue aortic	1.8	0.7	80	1.5

My final column "events" summarises and rounds the events and one could give this number to a patient, qualified by the statement that most are mild and recover.

From the same source we found that endocarditis risk was under 1% per annum.

45 When and how should a ventricular septal defect be closed in adults?

Seamus Cullen

Indications for surgical closure of a ventricular septal defect in childhood include congestive cardiac failure, pulmonary hypertension, severe aortic insufficiency and prior bacterial endocarditis. It is unlikely that a significant ventricular septal defect will be missed in childhood and therefore ventricular septal defects seen in adulthood tend to be small and isolated. In a small number of patients with Eisenmenger syndrome, i.e. ventricular septal defect with established pulmonary vascular disease, no intervention is possible.

The natural history of small congenital ventricular septal defects was thought to be favourable but longer follow up has demonstrated that 25% of adults with small ventricular septal defects may suffer from complications over longer periods of time. The complications documented were: infective endocarditis, aortic regurgitation, arrhythmias and myocardial dysfunction. Whilst closure of a ventricular septal defect protects against infective endocarditis, there are no data to suggest a protective effect against the development of late arrhythmias, sudden death or ventricular dysfunction.

The risk of bacterial endocarditis in patients with a ventricular septal defect is low (14.5 per 10,000 patient years). Prior or recurrent endocarditis on a ventricular septal defect would be deemed an indication for surgical closure even though the risks of endocarditis are low.

Whilst the majority of congenital ventricular septal defects are in the perimembranous or trabecular septum, a small percentage are found in the doubly committed subarterial position. This small sub group may be complicated by aortic valve cusp prolapse into the defect with development of subsequent aortic regurgitation which may be progressive and severe. The detection of aortic regurgitation in such a defect is considered an indication for surgical closure in most centres.

The mortality for surgical closure of a post-infarction ventricular septal defect may be up to 50%. Cardiogenic shock is exacerbated by the acute left ventricular volume load from the shunt through the ventricular septal defect. There is a small but growing experience of transcatheter device closure of such defects which avoids the need for cardiopulmonary bypass.

In summary, the indications for closure of a ventricular septal defect in an adult include the presence of a significant left to right shunt in the absence of pulmonary vascular disease, progressive aortic valve disease, recurrent endocarditis and acute post-infarction rupture in patients with haemodynamic compromise. Currently there is no evidence that closure of a small ventricular septal defect would prevent the occurrence of arrhythmias and ventricular dysfunction in the long term. The presence of established pulmonary vascular disease (Eisenmenger syndrome) is a contraindication to surgical intervention.

Further reading

Athanassiadi K, Apostolakis E, Kalavrouziotis G *et al*. Surgical repair of postinfarction ventricular septal defect: 10-year experience. *World J Surg* 1999;**23**: 64–7.

Backer CL, Winters RC, Zales VR *et al*. Restrictive ventricular septal defect: how small is too small to close? [See comments]. *Ann Thorac Surg* 1993;**56**: 1014–18.

Benton JP, Barker KS. Transcatheter closure of ventricular septal defect: a nonsurgical approach to the care of the patient with acute ventricular septal rupture. *Heart Lung* 1992;**21**: 356–64.

Kidd L, Driscoll DJ, Gersony WM *et al*. Second natural history study of congenital heart defects. Results of treatment of patients with ventricular septal defects. *Circulation* 1993;**87**: 138–51.

Neumayer U, Stone S, Somerville J. Small ventricular septal defects in adults. *Eur Heart J* 1998;**19**: 1573–82.

46 How should I treat atrial septal defects in adults?

Seamus Cullen

A significant secundum atrial septal defect (ASD) will result in volume and pressure overload of the right heart and may be associated with reduced exercise tolerance, shortness of breath and palpitations from atrial arrhythmias especially atrial fibrillation/flutter. Pulmonary vascular disease is a late complication, rarely seen before the fourth or fifth decade. The clinical suspicion of an ASD is confirmed by transoesophageal echocardiography as transthoracic images are usually inadequate. The presence of tricuspid regurgitation permits accurate assessment of right heart pressures, otherwise right heart catheterisation is required. Coronary angiography is indicated in patients over 40 years of age.

Indications for closure include symptoms (exercise intolerance, arrhythmias), right heart volume overload on echocardiography, the presence of a significant shunt (>2:1) or cryptogenic cerebrovascular events, especially associated with aneurysm of the oval foramen and right to left shunting demonstrated on contrast echocardiography during a Valsalva manoeuvre. Preoperative arrhythmias may persist after closure of the ASD but are associated with fewer symptoms. Reduction in left ventricular compliance due to e.g. hypertension/myocardial infarction will increase the left to right shunt through an ASD.

Closure of an ASD requires either surgery or transcatheter intervention. The results of surgery are excellent with little or no operative mortality in the absence of risk factors, e.g. pulmonary hypertension, co-morbidity. However, it requires a surgical scar, cardiopulmonary bypass and hospital stay of approximately 3–5 days. There is a small but definite risk of pericardial effusion with the potential for cardiac tamponade following closure of an atrial septal defect. The aetiology is poorly understood.

Transcatheter occlusion of ASDs is now established practice. Several occlusion devices are available. Their efficacy and ease of deployment have been demonstrated although long term data are lacking. It is possible to close ASDs with a stretched diameter of up to 34mm in size, providing there is a sufficient rim of atrial tissue. Our policy is to perform a transoesophageal echocardiogram under general anaesthesia with plans to proceed to device closure if the defect is suitable. Transoesophageal echocardiography is invaluable in guiding correct placement of the exposure. Heparin and antibiotics are administered during the procedure and intravenous heparinisation is used for the first 24 hours following deployment. Aspirin is administered for six weeks and then stopped, by which time the device will be covered by endothelial tissue. Mechanical problems seen with some earlier devices have not been encountered with the latest range. Medium term results have been encouraging.

Further reading
Berger F, Vogel M, Alexi-Meskishvili V *et al.* Comparison of results and complications of surgical and Amplatzer device closure of atrial septal defects. *J Thorac Cardiovasc Surg* 1999;**118**: 674–8.
Gatzoulis MA, Redington AN, Somerville J *et al.* Should atrial septal defects in adults be closed? *Ann Thorac Surg* 1996;**61**: 657–9.
Rigby ML. The era of transcatheter closure of atrial septal defects. *Heart* 1999;**81**: 227–8.

47 How do I follow up a patient who has had correction of aortic coarctation? What should I look for and how should they be managed?

Seamus Cullen

Long term follow up has demonstrated an increased cardio-vascular morbidity and mortality following repair of coarctation of the aorta. Repair at an older age has been associated with worse complications. Recoarctation may occur and produces upper body hypertension and pressure overload of the left ventricle. The type of surgical repair does not protect against recoarctation. Hypertension is a common complication affecting 8–20% of patients who have undergone repair of coarctation of the aorta and is associated with increased morbidity and mortality. It is associated with a later age at operation. Indeed, patients who are normotensive at rest may demonstrate an abnormally high increase in systolic blood pressure in response to exercise, probably related to baroreceptor abnormalities and/or reduced arterial compliance. The bicuspid aortic valve is commonly seen in patients with coarctation and may predispose to infective endocarditis, aortic stenosis/regurgitation and to ascending aortic aneurysm. In addition, mitral valve abnormalities have been detected in approximately 20% of patients.

All patients who have undergone repair of aortic coarctation should be followed up on a regular basis with careful monitoring of upper and lower limb blood pressure. Cardiac examination is directed towards palpation of the femoral pulses, monitoring of blood pressure and auscultation. Serial 12-lead ECG will detect the presence of left ventricular hypertrophy and annual transthoracic echocardiography is useful for screening for left ventricular hyper-trophy and recurrence of coarctation. A plain chest x-ray picture may demonstrate mediastinal widening related to aneurysm formation. However, magnetic resonance imaging is the gold standard for non-invasive diagnosis of recoarctation and/or aneurysm formation. Cardiac catheterisation confirms the presence of recoarctation and permits transcatheter balloon dilatation with stenting of the aortic coarctation. This is probably the procedure of choice in suitable lesions because of the small but definite risk of neurological complications associated with surgical correction of coarctation of the aorta. Persisting hypertension should be amenable to medical therapy, e.g. beta blockers providing aortic obstruction has been ruled out. Finally, patients who have had their coarctation repaired are at increased risk from infective endocarditis and antibiotic prophylaxis is recommended.

Further reading
Cohen M, Fuster V, Steele PM *et al.* Coarctation of the aorta. Long-term follow-up and prediction of outcome after surgical correction. *Circulation* 1989;**80**: 840–5.
Gardiner HM, Celermajer DS, Sorensen KE *et al.* Arterial reactivity is significantly impaired in normotensive young adults after successful repair of aortic coarctation in childhood. *Circulation* 1994;**89**: 1745–50.
Kaplan S, Perloff JK. Survival patterns after cardiac surgery or interventional catheterization: a broadening base. In: Perloff JK, Child JS. *Congenital heart disease in adults.* London and New York: W B Saunders Company, 1998.

48 How should I investigate a patient with hypertrophic cardiomyopathy (HCM)?

Krishna Prasad

The first step in the investigation of a patient with hypertrophic cardiomyopathy (HCM) is to establish the diagnosis and determine whether the case is sporadic or familial.

History

The investigation should begin with the taking of a *detailed history*. This should include the construction of a family tree with at least three generations.

The clinical examination

This should be aimed specifically at excluding other causes of hypertrophy such as aortic stenosis or hypertension.

Descriptive investigations

Electrocardiography. In the majority of patients, the 12-lead electrocardiogram (ECG) shows abnormalities such as voltage criteria for left ventricular hypertrophy (LVH), minor intraventricular conduction defects or bundle branch blocks. Only rarely (<5% of cases) is the ECG completely normal.

Echocardiography. The mainstay of diagnosis is the echocardiographic demonstration of left ventricular hypertrophy (LVH), with either the interventricular septum or the free wall measuring ≥15mm. A very detailed study by an experienced operator is often necessary as hypertrophy may involve any part of LV. It is important to note that for adults with family history of HCM, modified diagnostic criteria apply.

Investigations to identify risk factors of sudden death

The recognised risk factors are family history of sudden deaths, recurrent syncope, non-sustained ventricular tachycardia and an abnormal blood pressure response during exercise. History of multiple sudden deaths in the family is an important risk factor.

- *Ambulatory monitoring* of all patients with a diagnosis of HCM is mandatory and this should be for at least 48 hours.
- *Exercise electrocardiography* is also mandatory. Patients with HCM should undergo a metabolic exercise test with frequent blood pressure monitoring (every minute during exercise and for 5 minutes during recovery). An abnormal BP response is an important non-invasive marker of risk. The peak oxygen consumption during the exercise also helps identify those with significant limitation of exercise capacity.
- Non-sustained ventricular tachycardia ($\geq$5 beats rate of 120 beats) especially if repetitive, is also associated with increased risk of sudden death.

Additional investigations in patients with syncope

In these patients, additional investigations should be aimed at determining the mechanism.

- Repetitive Holter recordings should be made.
- Tilt table test and if necessary.
- Electrophysiological study to exclude accessory pathway.

Other investigations that may be useful but not mandatory

This includes electrophysiological studies and rarely a thallium scan for myocardial ischaemia. It is necessary to exclude significant coronary artery disease with a coronary angiogram in patients >40 years old, smokers or those with severe chest pain.

Reading list
Spirito P, Seidman CE, McKenna WJ *et al*. The management of hypertrophic cardiomyopathy. *N Engl J Med* 1997;**336**: 775–85.
McKenna WJ, Camm AJ. Sudden death in hypertrophic cardiomyopathy. Assessment of patients at high risk. *Circulation* 1989;**80**: 1489–92.
Maron BJ, Bonow RO, Cannon RO III *et al*. Hypertrophic cardiomyopathy. Interrelations of clinical manifestations, pathophysiology, and therapy(1). *N Engl J Med* 1987;**316**: 780–9.
Maron BJ, Bonow RO, Cannon RO III *et al*. Hypertrophic cardiomyopathy. Interrelations of clinical manifestations, pathophysiology, and therapy(2). *N Engl J Med* 1987;**316**: 844–52.

49 What is the medical therapy for patients with hypertrophic cardiomyopathy, and what surgical options are of use?

Krishna Prasad

About 40% of patients with hypertrophic cardiomyopathy (HCM) are symptomatic and a third have risk factors for sudden death. Each situation must be individually assessed. Asymptomatic patients do not need treatment routinely unless they are at risk of sudden death.

Treatment of symptoms

Typical symptoms include dyspnoea, palpitations and chest pain. Dyspnoea is usually due to left ventricular diastolic dysfunction while chest pain is frequently due to myocardial ischaemia. The pain may however be atypical and occur in the absence of demonstrable epicardial coronary disease. The treatment chosen will depend on whether there is significant outflow tract obstruction (outflow gradient ≥ 30mmHg). In those without obstruction, the choice is between either a beta blocker or a calcium antagonist, such as high dose verapamil (up to 480mg/day). In those with obstruction a beta blocker with or without disopyramide is usually the first choice for those patients with outflow obstruction (~25% of patients). Both drugs reduce the outflow gradient and improve diastolic function by their negative inotropism. Verapamil should only be used with caution as it may worsen the outflow obstruction (through the increased vasodilatation and consequent ventricular emptying with contraction). Palpitations may be due to supraventricular or ventricular arrhythmias. Supraventricular arrhythmias including atrial fibrillation may be controlled with beta blockers, verapamil or amiodarone.

Patients with refractory symptoms may be candidates for invasive treatment modalities such as dual chamber pacing with a short AV delay, alcohol septal ablation or surgical myectomy. Surgical septal myectomy is long established and can be combined with mitral valve replacement in patients with associated significant mitral regurgitation. When patients present with progressive ventricular dilatation and reduced systolic function, cardiac transplantation may need to be considered.

Prevention of sudden death

Identification and treatment of those at risk of sudden death is an important part of the management of patients with HCM. The known risk factors are family history of sudden death, recurrent syncope, non-sustained ventricular tachycardia and abnormal BP response during exercise. Patients with isolated risk factors need to be monitored carefully. Those with more than two risk factors clearly need treatment. Oral amiodarone and/or an implantable cardiac defibrillator are the available options.

Further reading

Seggewiss H, Gleichmann U, Faber L. Percutaneous transluminal septal myocardial ablation in hypertrophic obstructive cardiomyopathy: acute results and 3-month follow-up in 25 patients. *J Am Coll Cardiol* 1998;**31**: 252–8.

Spirito P, Seidman CE, McKenna WJ *et al*. The management of hypertrophic cardiomyopathy. *N Engl J Med* 1997 Mar 13;**336**: 775–85.

50 What is the role of permanent pacing in hypertrophic cardiomyopathy?

Niall G Mahon and W McKenna

There are broadly two categories of indications for permanent pace-maker insertion in patients with hypertrophic cardiomyopathy:

- Standard indications for pacing which apply to any patient.
- Reduction of left ventricular outflow tract gradient.

Indications for the use of dual chamber pacing with a short programmed atrioventricular delay for this purpose remain to be determined. Gradient reduction is thought to come about through a variety of effects on septal and papillary muscle motion and contractility. In general outflow gradients can be reduced by approximately 50% but the translation of this benefit into clinical improvement is variable and unpredictable. Initial enthusiasm has been tempered by equivocal results from clinical trials. A considerable placebo effect of the procedure has been observed in at least two randomised studies.[1,2] Anecdotally, patients who may benefit are symptomatic elderly patients with significant left ventricular outflow tract obstruction who do not respond to conventional therapy with beta blockers, verapamil or diso-pyramide. The role of pacing in young patients is unclear and methods of identifying patients likely to benefit from the procedure have not been established.

References
1 Nishimura RA, Trusty JM, Hayes DL *et al.* Dual chamber pacing for hypertrophic cardiomyopathy: a randomised double blind crossover trial. *J Am Coll Cardiol* 1997;**29**: 435–41.
2 Kappenberger L, Linde C, Daubert C *et al.* Pacing in hypertrophic obstructive cardiomyopathy. A randomised crossover study. PIC study group. *Eur Heart J* 1997;**18**: 1249–56.

Further reading
Elliott PM, Sharma S, McKenna WJ. Hypertrophic cardiomyopathy. In: Yusuf S, Cairns JA, Camm AJ *et al. Evidence based cardiology*. London: BMJ Books, 1998:722–43.

51 How do I investigate the relative of a patient with hypertrophic cardiomyopathy? How should they be followed up?

Niall G Mahon and W McKenna

Diagnostic criteria for the diagnosis of hypertrophic cardiomyopathy in first degree relatives have been proposed as shown in Table 51.1.

Table 51.1 Diagnostic criteria for the diagnosis of hypertrophic cardiomyopathy in first degree relatives

Major	Minor
Echocardiography	
Left ventricular wall thickness ≥13mm in the anterior septum or ≥15mm in the posterior septum or free wall	Left ventricular wall thickness of 12mm in the anterior septum or posterior wall or of 14mm in the posterior septum or free wall
Severe systolic anterior movement of the mitral valve leaflets (SAM) (causing septal leaflet contact)	Moderate SAM (no leaflet-septal contact)
	Redundant MV leaflets
Electrocardiography	
LVH + repolarisation changes	Complete BBB or minor interventricular conduction defect in LV leads
T wave inversion in leads I and aVL (≥3mm) (with QRS-T wave axis difference ≥30°), V3-V6 (≥3mm) or II and III and aVF(≥5mm)	Minor repolarisation changes in LV leads
Abnormal Q waves (>40ms or >25% R wave) in at least 2 leads from II, III, aVF (in the absence of left anterior hemiblock), V1-V4; or I, aVL, V5-V6	Deep S in V2 (>25mm)
	Unexplained syncope, chest pain dyspnoea

Source McKenna WJ, Spirito P, Desnos M *et al.* Experience from clinical genetics in hypertrophic cardiomyopathy. Proposal for new diagnostic criteria in adult members of affected families. *Heart* 1997;**77**: 130–2.

Hence first degree relatives should undergo history, physical examination, standard 2-D echocardiography, and 12-lead electrocardiography. Relatives are considered affected in the presence of one major criterion or two minor echocardiographic criteria or one minor echocardiographic plus two minor electro-cardiographic criteria. These criteria do not apply when other potential causes such as athletic training, systemic arterial hyper-tension or obesity are present. Young children with no evidence of disease should be re-evaluated every 5 years until their teens and then annually until aged 21. Diagnosis in a child under 10 years requires a body surface area corrected left ventricular wall thickness of >10mm. Affected relatives should additionally undergo risk stratification, which includes 48 hour Holter monitoring and exercise testing, looking especially for ventricular arrhythmias and abnormal blood pressure responses respectively.

Further reading
McKenna WJ, Spirito P, Desnos M *et al*. Experience from clinical genetics in hypertrophic cardiomyopathy. Proposal for new diagnostic criteria in adult members of affected families. *Heart* 1997;**77**: 130–2.

52 What investigation protocol should a patient with dilated cardiomyopathy undergo?

Niall G Mahon and W McKenna

A protocol for the investigation of dilated cardiomyopathy should aim to confirm the diagnosis, rule out treatable causes, prevent potential complications and determine prognosis. The following investigations are routinely used:

1 *Echocardiography.* Two-dimensional echocardiography is the major diagnostic test. Cardiac dimensions and systolic function are also of prognostic value, with an approximately 2-fold increase in relative risk of mortality for every 10% decline in ejection fraction.[1] The presence of intracardiac thrombi, as well as poor systolic function itself, may be indications for anticoagulation.
2 *Electrocardiography.* Twelve-lead electrocardiography and Holter monitoring for arrhythmias should be performed. Occasionally a diagnosis of incessant tachycardia as a cause of the cardiomyopathy may be made. The signal averaged ECG may be a useful predictor of risk of sudden death and progressive heart failure and should be performed where available.[2, 3]
3 *Metabolic exercise testing* is of prognostic value, particularly in advanced disease, and may guide referral for cardiac transplantation.
4 *Screens for metabolic causes* should routinely include liver function tests for unsuspected alcohol excess, thyroid function tests and iron studies including transferrin saturations. Further investigation (such as for sarcoid or amyloid) should be guided by history and examination.

Other tests may also be performed, but are not indicated in every case:

1 *Coronary angiography* should be performed in patients over the age of 40 years, or who have risk factors or symptoms or signs suggestive of coronary disease.
2 *Coxsackie and adenoviral titres* should be tested where there is a history of recent suspected myocarditis or recent viral illness, but the value of these in established cardiomyopathy is questionable.

3 *Serology* may be performed to detect the presence of markers of myocardial inflammation and myocyte damage.

4 *Endomyocardial biopsy* may have a role, but the risks and benefits are debated. What is, however, clear is that a tissue histological diagnosis provides important prognostic information which may (as in the case of sarcoidosis) have an impact on treatment.[4] Biopsy may be recommended to exclude treatable causes such as sarcoidosis and giant cell myocarditis, if these are thought likely. In research centres, biopsy specimens may be analysed by immunohistochemical and molecular biological techniques to determine the presence or absence of low grade inflammation and viral persistence.

Frequency of follow up will depend on the severity of involvement at initial presentation. The course of the disease at early follow up is a useful indicator of long term prognosis with improvement or deterioration occurring in most cases within six months to one year of diagnosis.

The possibility that the patient's cardiomyopathy may be familial should be explored by taking a detailed family history, but incomplete and age-related penetrance make family screening problematic. The decision to evaluate (usually first degree) relatives should be individualised, based on the extent of disease within a family, the levels of anxiety among patients and relatives, the presence of suggestive symptoms and the extent of local experience in the evaluation of dilated cardiomyopathy.

References

1 Sugrue DD, Rodeheffer RJ, Codd MB *et al*. The clinical course of idiopathic dilated cardiomyopathy. A population-based study. *Ann Intern Med* 1992;**117**: 117–23.

2 Mancini DM, Fleming K, Britton N, Simson MB. Predictive value of abnormal signal-averaged electrocardiograms in patients with nonischemic cardiomyopathy. *J Am Coll Cardiol* 1992;**19**: 72A.

3 Yi G, Keeling PJ, Goldman JH. *et al*. Comparison of time domain and spectral turbulence analysis of the signal-averaged electrocardiogram for the prediction of prognosis in idiopathic dilated cardiomyopathy. *Clin Cardiol* 1996;**19**: 800–8.

4 Felker GM, Thompson RE, Hare JM *et al*. Underlying causes and long-term survival in patients with initially unexplained cardiomyopathy. *N Engl J Med* 2000;**342**: 1077–84.

Further reading
Dec GW, Fuster V. Idiopathic dilated cardiomyopathy (review). *N Engl J Med* 1994;**331**: 1564–75.

53 Which patients with impaired ventricles should receive an ACE inhibitor? What are the survival advantages? Do AT1-receptor antagonists confer the same advantages?

Lionel H Opie

Not all impaired left ventricular (LV) function is an indication for ACE-inhibitor treatment. Specifically, left ventricular hypertrophy due to hypertension or aortic stenosis may be associated with diastolic dysfunction, yet ACE inhibition is only one of several therapies that will regress LV hypertrophy, even though some believe that for this purpose it is one of the best. Similarly, the defects of ventricular function seen in hypertrophic cardiomyopathy are not a clear indication for ACE inhibition.

The following patients *should* be treated with an ACE inhibitor

Symptomatic patients

All patients with clinically diagnosed heart failure should receive an ACE inhibitor. The survival advantages are consistent (mortality reduction of about 20%) and far outweigh the relatively small risk of serious side effects. In post-infarct clinically diagnosed heart failure, ACE inhibition reduced mortality by 27% at an average follow up of 15 months, and 36% with a mean follow up of nearly 5 years.[1]

Post-infarct patients without overt heart failure but with impaired left ventricular systolic function

These patients should receive an ACE inhibitor. This will give them benefit even in the absence of symptoms, as shown in the SOLVD prevention trial.[2] Most patients were post-infarct, and most were New York Heart Association (NYHA) class 1, despite the low ejection fraction of 35% or less.

Benefit to risk ratios

In the SAVE study[3] of post-infarct patients with an ejection fraction of ≤40%, the chief treatment-related adverse effects of captopril were cough, taste abnormally, dizziness or hypotension. Calculations suggest that a reduction in mortality could be achieved without side effects after treating only 24 patients.[4] Yet nearly 200 patients would have to be treated before encountering one case in which side effects were found without a mortality benefit. This makes ACE inhibition a very safe form of therapy.

Do AT1-receptor blockers confer the same advantages?

These agents are not currently (1999) licenced for use in heart failure in the USA nor in the UK. There are some key theoretical differences from ACE inhibitors, such as decreased breakdown of the protective vasodilator bradykinin during ACE inhibition, versus the likelihood that AT1 blockade gives more complete inhibition of the renin-angiotensin system than does ACE inhibition. The ELITE II trial showed losartan to be no more effective than captopril in reducing mortality in the elderly. In the subgroup of patients taking beta blockers, mortality decreased in those taking captopril, compared with losartan. ACE inhibitors, therefore, remain the cornerstone of the therapy of heart failure.[5]

It should be noted that data support the use of spironolactone administration (25mg/day) in those with severe heart failure. Concerns about hyperkalaemia relating to concomitant use with ACE inhibition were generally unfounded in this study, although potassium levels in the order of 6mmol/l were accepted.[6]

References

1 Hall AS, Murray GD, and Ball SG. Follow-up study of patients randomly allocated ramipril or placebo for heart failure after acute myocardial infarction: AIRE Extension (AIREX) Study. Acute Infarction Ramipril Efficacy. *Lancet* 1997;**349**: 1493–7.

2 The SOLVD Investigators. Effects of enalapril on mortality and the development of heart failure in asymptomatic patients with reduced left ventricular ejection fractions. *N Engl J Med.* 1992;**327**: 685–91.

3 Pfeffer MA, Braunwald E, Moye LA *et al*. Effect of captopril on mortality and morbidity in patients with left ventricular dysfunction after myocardial infarction. Results of the survival and ventricular enlargement trial. *N Engl J Med* 1992;**327**: 669–77.

4 Mancini GB, Schulzer M. Reporting risks and benefits of therapy by use of the concepts of unqualified success and unmitigated failure: applications to highly cited trials in cardiovascular medicine. *Circulation* 1999;**99**: 377–83.

5 Topol E. ACE inhibitors still the drug of choice for heart failure – and more. *Lancet* 1999;**354**: 1797.
6 Pitt B, Zannad F, Remme WJ *et al*. The effect of spironolactone on morbidity and mortality in patients with severe heart failure. Randomized Aldactone Evaluation Study Investigators. *N Engl J Med* 1999;**341**: 709–17.

54 What is the role of vasodilators in chronic heart failure? Who should receive them?

Lionel H Opie

There are three main groups of vasodilator therapies used in the treatment of chronic heart failure.

Nitrates alone

Nitrates on their own can be used intermittently for relief of dyspnoea – not well documented, but logical to try. For example, intermittent sublingual or oral nitrates may benefit a patient already on high doses of loop diuretics and an ACE inhibitor, but who still has severe exertional or nocturnal dyspnoea, and needs relief. The continuous use of nitrates does, however, run the risk of nitrate tolerance, which in turn may be lessened by combination with hydralazine.[1]

Nitrates plus hydralazine

Nitrates plus hydralazine are better than placebo in chronic heart failure, although inferior to ACE inhibitors. They therefore represent treatment options when the patient experiences ACE intolerance, although the drugs of choice for this situation would be the angiotensin receptor blockers.

The long-acting dihydropyridines (DHPs, e.g. amlodipine and felodipine)

Regarding the calcium blockers, the non-DHPs are contra-indicated whereas the long acting DHP amlodipine has suggestive benefit on mortality in non-ischemic cardiomyopathy, as shown in the PRAISE study.[2] In the ischaemic patients, the drug was safe yet without any suggestion of mortality benefit. Hypothetically, part of the benefit in dilated cardiomyopathy could be by inhibition of cytokine production,[3] and not by vasodilatation. PRAISE 2 is focusing on non-ischaemic cardiomy-opathy patients. In the meantime, long acting DHPs such as amlodipine or felodipine may be cautiously added when heart failure patients still have angina that persists after nitrates and beta blockade, or hypertension despite ACE inhibitors, beta blockers and diuretics. Yet with the convincing evidence for real benefits from beta blockade in heart failure, the DHPs should probably only be used, even for these limited indications, if beta blockade is contraindicated.

The inotropic dilators ("inodilators") such as amrinone and milrinone are very useful in acute heart failure, but are not safe in chronic heart failure, as warned by the FDA because of the risks of increased hospitalisation and mortality.[4]

References

1 Gogia H, Mehra A, Parikh S *et al.* Prevention of tolerance to hemo-dynamic effects of nitrates with concomitant use of hydralazine in patients with chronic heart failure. *J Am Coll Cardiol* 1995;**26**: 1575–80.

2 Packer M, O'Connor CM, Ghali JK *et al.* Effect of amlodipine on morbidity and mortality in severe chronic heart failure. Prospective Randomized Amlodipine Survival Evaluation Study Group. *N Engl J Med* 1996;**335**: 1107–14.

3 Mohler ER, Sorensen LC, Ghali JK *et al.* Role of cytokines in the mech-anism of action of amlodipine: the PRAISE Heart Failure Trial. Prospective Randomized Amlodipine Survival Evaluation. *J Am Coll Cardiol* 1997;**30**: 35–41.

4 Thadani U, Roden DM. FDA Panel Report. *Circulation* 1998;**97**: 2295–6.

55 Should I give digoxin to patients with heart failure if they are in sinus rhythm? If so, to whom? Are there dangers to stopping it once started?

Lionel H Opie

This is a very contentious issue. It is well known that the only prospective trial that was powered for mortality, failed to show that digoxin could lessen deaths.[1] On the other hand, hospitalisation from all causes, including cardiovascular, was reduced by 6%. Personally, bearing in mind all the hazards of digoxin, I would rather add to the basic diuretic-ACE inhibitor therapy, spironolactone in a low dose (25mg daily). The latter improves mortality substantially, as shown in the RALES study.[2]

Or, if I had the patience and skill, and the patient is haemodynamically stable, I would add a beta blocker such as bisoprolol, metoprolol or carvedilol, starting in a very low dose given to a haemodynamically stable patient and working up the dose over 2 to 3 months. Any doubt about the mortality benefit of beta blockade has been removed by the recent CIBIS study.[3] If after all this I was still looking for further improvement, I would certainly add digoxin but take great care to avoid overdosing, which can be fatal, especially in the presence of a low plasma potassium level. Once I had started digoxin, I would not hesitate to stop it if toxicity were suspected. But if the patient came to me already taking digoxin with a low therapeutic blood level, and seemed to be doing well, then I would not stop the drug. The problems with digoxin withdrawal suggested by the withdrawal trials such as RADIANCE is that they merely show that patients who do well while on digoxin, should not have it withdrawn.[4] These are non-randomised trials and give no information on how the patients reacted to the addition of digoxin. For example, to take an extreme case, if digoxin had potentially adverse effects, and actually killed patients, such an increase of mortality could not be detected by assessing the effects of withdrawal of the drug from the survivors.

References

1 The effect of digoxin on mortality and morbidity in patients with heart failure. The Digitalis Investigation Group. *N Engl J Med* 1997;**336**: 525–33.

2 Pitt B, Zannad F, Remme WJ *et al.* for the Randomized Aldactone Evaluation Study Investigators (RALES). The effect of spironolactone on morbidity and mortality in patients with severe heart failure. *N Engl J Med* 1999;**341**: 709–17.
3 The Cardiac Insufficiency Bisoprolol Study II (CIBIS-II): a randomised trial. *Lancet* 1999;**353**: 9–13.
4 Packer M, Gheorghiade M, Young JB *et al.* Withdrawal of digoxin from patients with chronic heart failure treated with angiotensin-converting-enzyme inhibitors. RADIANCE Study. *N Engl J Med* 1993;**329**: 1–7.

56 Which patients with heart failure should have a beta blocker? How do I start it and how should I monitor therapy?

Rakesh Sharma

More than 25 years ago it was proposed that beta blockers may be of benefit in heart failure[1] and yet, until recently, there has been a general reluctance amongst the medical profession to prescribe them for this indication. This is not entirely surprising, as not too long ago heart failure was widely considered to be a major contraindication for the use of beta blockers. There is now considerable evidence from major clinical trials that beta blockers are capable of improving both the symptoms and prognosis of patients with congestive heart failure (CHF).

The results from the second Cardiac Insufficiency Bisoprolol Study (CIBIS-II) and the Metoprolol CR/XL Randomised Intervention Trial in Heart Failure (MERIT-HF) have shown that selective β1 antagonists (i.e. bisoprolol and metoprolol respectively) can improve survival in patients with CHF.[2,3] Carvedilol, a relatively new agent, is a non-selective beta blocker, which also has antioxidant effects and causes vasodilatation. A multi-centre US study showed there to be a 65% mortality reduction with carvedilol as compared with placebo.[4] At present it is not clear whether β1 selectivity is important with respect to therapy in CHF, and this question is currently being addressed in the Carvedilol and Metoprolol European Trial (COMET).

In the UK, carvedilol has been licensed for the treatment of mild to moderate CHF (NYHA class II or III) and bisoprolol is also likely to be approved in the near future. Prior to commencement with beta blockers, patients should be clinically stable and maintained on standard therapy with diuretics, ACE inhibitors +/– digoxin. There is insufficient evidence at present to recommend the treatment of unstable or NYHA class IV patients. The Carvedilol Prospective Randomised Cumulative Survival Trial (COPERNICUS), which is recruiting patients with severe CHF, (NYHA class IIIB-IV) will hopefully be able to answer this question in the future.

Treatment should be initiated at a low dose and be increased gradually under supervised care. The patient should be monitored for 2–3 hours after the initial dose and after each subsequent dose increase to ensure that there is no deterioration in symptoms, significant bradycardia, or hypotension. In patients with suspected or known renal impairment, it is recommended that serum biochemistry is also monitored. A suggested protocol is as follows: initiate carvedilol at 3.125mg twice daily; the dose may be doubled at intervals of two weeks to a maximum of 25mg twice daily, depending upon tolerance.

It is clear that beta blockers are of prognostic benefit in patients with stable CHF who are in NYHA class II to III. However, there are several important areas in which the effect of beta blocker therapy is unknown. For example, should we be using beta blockers to treat asymptomatic patients with evidence of systolic ventricular dysfunction and is there a role for beta blocker therapy in the patient post-myocardial infarction who has ventricular impairment? Clinical trials are currently being performed to answer these questions.

Evidence of a beneficial effect of beta blockers on the syndrome of heart failure is accumulating. The use of beta blockers in this context may prove to be one of the most important pharmacological "re-discoveries" in cardiology in recent years.

References
1 Swedberg K. History of beta-blockers in congestive heart failure. *Heart* 1998;**79**: S29–30.
2 The Cardiac Insufficiency Bisoprolol Study II (CIBIS-II): a randomised trial. *Lancet* 1999;**353**: 9–13.
3 Effect of metoprolol CR/XL in chronic heart failure: Metoprolol CR/XL Randomised Intervention Trial in Congestive Heart Failure (MERIT-HF). *Lancet* 1999;**353**: 2001–7.
4 Packer M, Colucci WS, Sackner-Bernstein JD *et al.* Double-blind, placebo-controlled study of the effects of carvedilol in patients with moderate to severe heart failure. The PRECISE Trial. Prospective Randomized Evaluation of Carvedilol on Symptoms and Exercise. *Circulation* 1996;**94**: 2793–9.

57 What is mean and model life expectancy in NYHA I-IV heart failure?

Aidan Bolger

The New York Heart Association (NYHA) first published its *Criteria for diagnosis and treatment of heart disease* in 1928. The ninth and latest edition, published in 1994,[1] retains an assessment of the functional capacity of the patient with heart disease (see Table 57.1). The NYHA functional capacity score is an entirely subjective assessment of a patient's cardiovascular status and is independent of objective measures of cardiovascular structure and function. Despite this it remains a quick, simple and reproducible evaluation of the patient with heart failure. In testament to this, NYHA class can consistently predict mortality in chronic heart failure having now been established as an independent prognostic variable in this condition in many large, epidemiological studies and clinical trials. The majority of patients with class IV functional status have end stage disease, the poorest prognosis and represent a relatively small group. Most patients are therefore classified with class II or III symptoms. Larger studies have reported mortality data across all NYHA classes. Typically the mortality rates for one and three years respectively are, class I/II 82% and 52%, class III 77% and 34% and class IV 41% and 0%.[2]

Hospital series include those with acutely decompensated disease. Whether such patients can be classified according to NYHA criteria is open to debate, but they might be considered in class IV. Survival of just 33% at two year follow up has been reported for this group in a Canadian study.[3] The burden of heart failure in the United Kingdom is more difficult to appreciate, based on the analysis of official surveys, as death certification is based on disease aetiology rather than clinical diagnoses.

The Framingham Heart Study[4] is probably the largest survey of cardiovascular disease undertaken and has data on over 9000 patients, spanning two generations, with a median follow up of 14.8 years. Mortality data in this series was not based on NYHA class but simply included those in which a diagnosis of heart failure had been made. The overall five year mortality rates were reported as 75% for men and 62% for women with a median survival of 1.66 years after the onset of congestive heart failure.

After excluding the patients who died within 90 days of diagnosis (likely to contain many with NYHA class IV disease) the mortality rates fell to 65% for men and 47% for women. The authors of this study[4] emphasise the grim prognosis of this disease by making comparison to the mortality rate for all cancers, which, between 1979 and 1984 was reported as 50%.

The overall prognosis for a patient diagnosed with heart failure is therefore really rather wretched. The application of the NYHA functional score provides a simple but meaningful way of stratifying such patients to help formulate management priorities. Many objective prognostic variables with equal or greater weight in predicting heart failure mortality have been elucidated,[5] however, and account of these should be acknowledged.

Table 57.1   New York Heart Association classification of functional capacity in patients with cardiac disease

NYHA class	Functional capacity
I	Patients with cardiac disease, but without resulting limitation of physical activity. Ordinary physical activity does not cause undue fatigue, palpitation, dyspnea, or anginal pain.
II	Patients with cardiac disease resulting in slight limitation of physical activity. They are comfortable at rest. Ordinary physical activity results in fatigue, palpitation, dyspnea, or anginal pain.
III	Patients with marked limitation of physical activity. They are comfortable at rest. Less than ordinary activity causes fatigue, palpitation, dyspnea, or anginal pain.
IV	Patients with cardiac disease resulting in inability to carry on any physical activity without discomfort. Symptoms of heart failure or of the anginal syndrome may be present even at rest. If any physical activity is undertaken, discomfort is increased.

References

1 The Criteria Committee of the New York Heart Association. Criteria for diagnosis and treatment of heart disease, 9th edition, Little, Brown and Company, 1994.
2 Keogh AM, Baron DW, Hickie JB. Prognostic guides in patients with idiopathic or ischemic dilated cardiomyopathy assessed for cardiac transplantation. *Am J Cardiol* 1990;**65**: 903–8.

3 Brophy JM, Deslauriers G, Rouleau JL. Long-term prognosis of patients presenting to the emergency room with decompensated congestive heart failure. *Can J Cardiol* 1994;**10**: 543–7.

4 Ho KK, Anderson KM, Kannel WB, Grossman W, Levy D. Survival after the onset of congestive heart failure in Framingham Heart Study subjects. *Circulation* 1993;**88**: 107–15.

5 Cowburn PJ, Cleland JG, Coats AJ, Komajda M. Risk stratification in chronic heart failure. *Eur Heart J* 1998;**19**: 696–710.

58 What are LVADs and BIVADS, and who should have them?

Brendan Madden

Over the past 30 years, there have been efforts to produce a mechanical device that can replace the human heart. Extracorporeal univentricular and biventricular implantable devices are available, which can support the failing heart following conventional cardiac surgery, or while awaiting transplantation. The number of potential recipients already far exceeds the number of available donor organs, however, and temporary holding measures that increase the size of the recipient pool only increase the number of patients that die awaiting transplantation.

Devices available include:

- Left Ventricular Assist Device (LVAD)
- Right Ventricular Assist Device (RVAD)
- Biventricular Assist Devices (BIVADS)

At present they are used for selected patients as a bridge to transplantation or occasionally to support patients with cardiomyopathy or myocarditis or those who cannot be successfully weaned from cardiopulmonary bypass following conventional cardiac surgical procedures. An LVAD or RVAD is used depending on which ventricle is failing. These devices consist of extracorporeal pumps, which remove blood from the atria bypassing the ventricles, and deliver it to the aorta and pulmonary circulation. The output of each assist device can be gradually reduced if the patient's heart recovers. Indeed, in some patients, successful weaning from artificial circulatory support has been described. Others have been successfully bridged to cardiac transplantation using an assist device. These devices are, however, expensive. They are associated with numerous complications, which include infection with Aspergillus species, haematological complications and multiple organ failure. It is not yet known whether the devices are sufficiently free of long term complications to be an effective treatment modality.

Further reading

Elbeery JR, Owen CH, Savitt MA *et al*. Effects of the left ventricular assist device on right ventricular function. *J Thorac Cardiovasc Surg* 1990;**99**: 809–16.

Kormos RL, Borovetz HS, Gasior T *et al*. Experience with univentricular support in mortally ill cardiac transplant candidates. *Ann Thorac Surg* 1990;**49**: 261–72.

59 Who is eligible for a heart or heart-lung transplant? How do I assess suitability for transplantation?

Brendan Madden

Cardiac and pulmonary transplantation are potential options for selected patients with end stage cardiac or pulmonary disease, unresponsive to conventional medical or surgical therapies. The majority of patients referred for cardiac transplantation have end stage cardiac failure as a consequence of ischaemic heart disease or cardiomyopathy, although some patients are referred whose cardiac failure follows valvular or congenital heart disease. There are four lung transplant procedures, namely, heart-lung transplantation, bilateral lung transplantation, single lung transplantation and living related lobar transplantation.

With increasing numbers of centres performing cardiac transplantation worldwide, fewer combined heart-lung transplant procedures are being performed. Therefore, the indications for this operation have been redefined and by and large, heart and lung transplantation is now reserved for patients with Eisenmenger syndrome who have a surgically incorrectable cardiac defect. Broadly speaking, patients with suppurative lung disease, e.g. cystic fibrosis and bronchiectasis, require bilateral lung transplantation. Single lung transplantation is usually inappropriate for this group because of the concern of contamination of the allograft from sputum overspill from the native remaining lung in an immunocompromised patient. Single lung transplantation has been successfully applied to patients with end stage respiratory failure due to restrictive lung conditions, e.g. pulmonary fibrosis, and to selected patients with emphysema. In living related lobar transplantation a lower lobe is taken from two living related donors, the transplant recipient undergoes bilateral pneumonectomy and subsequent re-implantation of a lower lobe into each hemithorax. Encouraging results for this procedure have been described in adolescents with cystic fibrosis.

Cardiac transplantation – indications

1 Prognosis less than 12 months
2 Inability to lead a satisfactory life because of physical limitation caused by cardiac failure

3 New York Heart Association class III or IV
4 Non-transplant cardiac surgery considered unfeasible
5 Heart failure resulting from one of the following:
- Ischaemic heart disease
- Cardiomyopathy
- Valvular heart disease
- Congenital heart disease.

Lung transplantation – indications

1 Severe respiratory failure, despite maximal medical therapy
2 Severely impaired quality of life
3 Patient positively wants a transplant.

Only patients who have deteriorating chronic respiratory failure should be accepted on to the transplant waiting list. In practice, the forced expiratory volume in one second is usually less than 30% of the predicted value.

Careful psychological assessment is necessary to exclude patients with intractable psychosocial instability that may interfere with their ability to cope with the operation and to comply with the strict post operative follow up and immuno-suppressive regimes. In most centres, the upper age limit is 60 years for cardiac transplantation and for single lung transplantation and 50 years for heart-lung and bilateral lung transplantation.

Contraindications for cardiac and lung transplantation

1 Psychosocial instability and poor compliance
2 Infection with hepatitis B or C virus or with human immuno-deficiency virus
3 Active mycobacterial or aspergillus infection
4 Active malignancy (patient must be in complete remission for more than five years after treatment)
5 Active peptic ulceration
6 Severe osteoporosis
7 Other end-organ failure not amenable to transplantation e.g. hepatic failure or renal failure (creatinine clearance <50mls/min).

Incremental risk factors for pulmonary transplantation include previous thoracic surgery and pleurodesis and patients are not accepted on to the waiting list who are on long term prednisolone therapy in excess of 10mg/d. Additional contraindications for cardiac transplantation include pulmonary vascular resistance greater than 3 Wood units and severe lung disease.

Further reading
Madden B. Lung transplantation. In: Hodson MR, Geddes DM, eds. *Cystic fibrosis*. London: Chapman & Hall, 1994: 329–46.
Madden B, Geddes D. Which patients should receive lung transplants? *Monaldi Arch Chest Dis* 1993;**48:** 346–52.
Murday AJ, Madden BP. Surgery for heart and lung failure. *Surgery* 1996;**14:** 18–24

---

128 — 100 Questions in Cardiology

60 What are the survival figures for heart and heart-lung transplantation?

Brendan Madden

In the International Registry for Heart and Lung Transplantation, the one year actuarial survival following cardiac transplantation is approximately 80%. Thereafter there is an annual attrition rate of 2 to 4% so that five year actuarial survival and ten year actuarial survival is approximately 65% and 50% respectively. One and three year actuarial survival following heart-lung and bilateral lung transplantation is approximately 70% and 50% respectively and approximately 80% and 60% respectively following single lung transplantation. Most survivors demonstrate a marked improvement in quality of life. Lung function increases rapidly following surgery and forced expiratory volume in one second and forced vital capacity are usually in excess of 70% by the end of the third postoperative month. Results of living related lobar transplantation are similar to those for heart-lung and bilateral lung transplantation.

The most serious late complication following cardiac transplantation is transplant associated coronary artery disease and following pulmonary transplantation is obliterative bronchiolitis.

Further reading

Madden B, Hodson M, Tsang V *et al.* Intermediate term results of heart-lung transplantation for cystic fibrosis. *Lancet* 1992;**339**: 1583–7.

Madden B, Radley-Smith R, Hodson M *et al.* Medium term results of heart and lung transplantation. *J Heart Lung Transplant* 1992;**11**: S241–3.

Murday AJ, Madden BP. Surgery for heart and lung failure. *Surgery* 1996;**14**: 18–24.

61 What drugs do post-transplant patients require, and what are their side effects? How should I follow up such patients?

Brendan Madden

Following successful cardiac, cardiopulmonary or pulmonary transplantation, patients require life-long immunosuppressive therapy. Routine immunosuppression consists of cyclosporin-A and azathioprine, occasionally supplemented by cortico-steroids. Episodes of acute allograft rejection are treated with intravenous methylprednisolone therapy or occasionally anti-thymocyte globulin or OKT3. Other drugs used include tacrolimus, mycophenolate mofetil and cyclophosphamide. Early evidence suggests that mycophenolate mofetil (an antimetabolite drug) may be a useful alternative to azathioprine as maintenance postoperative immunosuppression. OKT3 is a monoclonal antibody raised in mice, which is directed against the lymphocyte CD3 complex. Although it is sometimes used for induction following transplantation it is now more frequently employed in the management of severe episodes of acute cardiac rejection.

Common complications following transplantation include allograft rejection and infection. It is of paramount importance to immunosuppress the patient to minimise the risk of allograft rejection, without over-immunosuppressing and thereby increasing susceptibility to opportunistic infection. For this reason, cyclosporin-A blood levels are regularly monitored post-operatively. Side effects include renal failure, hypertension, hyperkalaemia, hirsutism, gum hypertrophy and increased susceptibility to opportunistic infection and to lympho-proliferative disorders. Tacrolimus acts in a similar way to cyclosporin-A although it may be a more potent immunosup-pressive agent. Although its side effect profile is similar, diabetes mellitus can be a complication. Azathioprine is an antimetabolite whose major side effects include bone marrow suppression and hepatic cholestasis. Occasionally pancreatitis can occur. Some patients who are intolerant of azathioprine are prescribed mycophenolate mofetil (which is less likely to cause bone marrow suppression) or cyclophosphamide. At the present time the precise role of tacrolimus and mycophenolate in post-cardiac and pulmonary transplant immunosuppression is unclear and requires further study. The side effect profile of corticosteroid therapy is well documented.

In addition to regular monitoring of drug levels and haematological (full blood count) and biochemical (renal and hepatic function, blood glucose) indices, one should be aware of drug interactions which may reduce or increase the levels or effectiveness of immunosuppressive agents. For example drugs which promote hepatic enzyme induction (e.g. anticonvulsants, antituberculous therapy) will reduce cyclosporin-A levels. Certain antibiotics (e.g. erythromycin) and calcium channel blockers (e.g. diltiazem) will increase cyclosporin-A levels. Similar interactions apply to tacrolimus. Non-steroidal anti-inflammatory agents can potentiate nephrotoxicity when given with cyclosporin-A or tacrolimus. The dose of azathioprine has to be reduced by 70% if patients are also prescribed allopurinol.

Further reading

Madden B. Late complications following cardiac transplantation. *Br Heart J* 1994;**72**: 89–91.

Madden B, Kamalvand K, Chan CM *et al*. The medical management of patients with cystic fibrosis following heart-lung transplantation. *Eur Resp J* 1993;**6**: 965–70.

Madden BP. Immunocompromise and opportunistic infection in organ transplantation. *Surgery* 1998;**16**: 37–40.

62 Can a cardiac transplant patient get angina? How is this investigated?

Brendan Madden

Post-transplant cardiac denervation theoretically abolishes the perception of cardiac chest pain. However, some patients may develop postoperative typical anginal chest pain precipitated by exercise or by increasing heart rate. This has been associated with ECG evidence of ischaemia and coronary angiography has confirmed transplant associated coronary artery disease. Such symptoms, however, are usually described by patients who are more than five years following transplantation. Chest pain associated with coronary artery disease is uncommon in patients who are less than five years post-cardiac transplantation. Interestingly, recent evidence shows an absence of bradycardic response to apnoea and hypoxia in cardiac transplant recipients with obstructive sleep apnoea. It may be that prospective overnight polysomnography studies will identify parasympathetic re-innervation in this group.

The majority of patients with transplant associated coronary artery disease do not get chest pain. Presenting features include progressive dyspnoea with exertion or the signs and symptoms of cardiac failure. Cardiac auscultation may reveal a third or fourth heart sound or features of heart failure. The ECG may show rhythm disturbances or a reduction in total voltage (the summation of the R and S wave in leads I, II, III, V1 and V6). Transthoracic 2D echocardiography may reveal evidence of poor biventricular function. Most units do not advocate routine annual coronary angiography for asymptomatic patients, since the angiographic findings do not usually alter clinical managment. Furthermore, conventional coronary angiography does not always confirm the diagnosis; intravascular ultrasound may be more sensitive. The condition is frequently diffuse and distal and not usually amenable to intervention, e.g. with angioplasty, stent insertion or bypass surgery. In those patients who have a localised lesion, the disease may progress despite successful intervention. The majority of centres do not usually offer cardiac re-transplantation on account of shortage of donor organs and poor results attendant on cardiac re-transplantation. Therefore patients who develop this condition are usually managed medically.

Further reading

Grant SCD, Brooks NH. Accelerated graft atherosclerosis after heart transplantation. *Br Heart J* 1993;**69**: 469–70.

Madden B, Shenoy V, Dalrymple-Hay M *et al.* Absence of bradycardic response to apnoea and hypoxia in cardiac transplant recipients with obstructive sleep apnoea. *J Heart Lung Transplant* 1997;**16**: 394–7.

Mann J. Graft vascular disease in heart transplant patients. *Br Heart J* 1992;**68**: 253–4.

63 What drugs should be used to maintain someone in sinus rhythm who has paroxysmal atrial fibrillation? Is there a role for digoxin?

Suzanna Hardman and Martin Cowie

The natural history of patients with paroxysmal atrial fibrillation is that over a period of time (and often many years) there is a gradual tendency to an increased frequency and duration of attacks. A proportion of patients will develop chronic atrial fibrillation. Not all patients require antiarrhythmic drugs and the potential side effects and inconvenience of regular medication must be balanced against the frequency of episodes and symptomatology which vary markedly between patients. Triggers include alcohol and caffeine, ischaemia, untreated hypertension (which if aggressively managed can at least in the short term obviate the need for antiarrhythmics), thyrotoxicosis, and in a small proportion of patients vagal or sympathetic stimulation where attacks are typically preceded by a drop in heart rate or exercise respectively.

The most effective drugs are also those with potentially dangerous side effects. The risks of class 1 agents (such as flecainide, disopyramide and propafenone) in patients with underlying coronary artery disease are well recognised and are best avoided. In younger patients (where it is presumed the associated risks are proportionately less) they can be highly effective. Sotalol may be useful in some patients but adequate dosing is required to achieve class 3 antiarrhythmic activity and not all patients will tolerate the associated degree of beta blockade. Amiodarone can be highly effective but its use is limited by the incidence of serious side effects. Beta blockers and calcium channel blockers have no role in preventing paroxysms of atrial fibrillation but can help certain patients in reducing the rate and so symptomatology.

Despite the long-standing conviction of many clinicians that digoxin is efficacious in the management of paroxysmal atrial fibrillation it has been clearly shown that digoxin neither reduces the frequency of attacks nor produces any useful reduction of heart rate during paroxysms of atrial fibrillation. Furthermore a number of placebo-controlled studies designed to explore the possibility that digoxin might chemically cardiovert patients with recent onset atrial fibrillation have shown no effect of digoxin as compared with placebo. Hence there appears to be no role for digoxin.

Further reading

Falk RH, Knowlton AA, Bernard SA *et al*. Digoxin for converting recent-onset atrial fibrillation to sinus rhythm. *Ann Intern Med* 1987;**106**: 503–6.

Jordaens L, Trouerbach PC, Tavernier R *et al*. Conversion of atrial fibrillation to sinus rhythm and rate control by digoxin in comparison to placebo. *Eur Heart J* 1997;**18**: 643–8.

Rawles JM, Metcalfe MJ, Jennings K. Time of occurrence, duration, and ventricular rate of paroxysmal atrial fibrillation: the effect of digoxin. *Br Heart J* 1990;**63**: 224–7.

64 Which patients with paroxysmal or chronic atrial fibrillation should I treat with aspirin, warfarin or neither?

Suzanna Hardman and Martin Cowie

Patients in whom the risk of thromboembolism is considered to be greater than the risk of a serious bleed due to warfarin should be considered for formal anticoagulation. In published clinical trials of anticoagulation the risk of stroke was reduced from 4.3% per year to 1.3% per year with anticoagulation. This equates to 30 strokes prevented for 1000 patients treated with warfarin for 12 months. Whether such benefit can be seen in routine practice depends not only on a careful decision for each patient regarding the risk of bleeding and the risk of thromboembolism, but also on the quality of monitoring the intensity of anticoagulation. The usual practice is to anticoagulate to a target INR of 2.5 (range 2–3), unless there is a history of recurrent thromboemboli in which case higher intensity anticoagulation may be necessary. In the clinical trials the risk of serious bleeding was 0.9% per year in the control group and slightly higher (1.3%) in those on warfarin. Risk factors for bleeding on anticoagulants include serious co-morbid disease (such as anaemia, renal, cerebrovascular or liver disease), previous gastrointestinal bleeding, erratic or excessive alcohol misuse, uncontrolled hypertension, immobility, and poor quality clinical and anticoagulant monitoring.

Aspirin therapy is often recommended for elderly patients with atrial fibrillation on the basis that there is a lower risk of bleeding compared with warfarin. The likely benefits of aspirin are also less than those of warfarin. Further, the bulk of AF-associated stroke occurs in those aged >75 years, and the benefits of anti-coagulation are not outweighed by the risks in high-risk elderly patients in whom monitoring is carefully carried out.[1] Where warfarin is genuinely considered unsuitable (or is unacceptable to a patient), and the patient is at significant risk of thrombo-embolism, there is evidence that aspirin at a dose of 325mg per day reduces the risk of thromboembolism, but no evidence that lower doses are effective. The combination of fixed-dose low intensity warfarin with aspirin confers no benefit over conventional warfarin therapy in terms of bleeding risks and is less effective in preventing thromboembolism.

References
1 Hart RG. Warfarin in atrial fibrillation: underused in the elderly, often inappropriately used in the young. *Heart* 1999;**82**: 539–40.

Further reading
Stroke Prevention in Atrial Fibrillation Investigators. Adjusted dose warfarin versus low-intensity, fixed dose warfarin plus aspirin for high-risk patients with atrial fibrillation: stroke prevention in atrial fibrillation III. *Lancet* 1996;**348**: 633–8.
Stroke Prevention In Atrial Fibrillation Investigators. Stroke Prevention in Atrial Fibrillation Study. Final results. *Circulation* 1991;**84**: 527–39.
Hardman SM, Cowie M. Fortnightly review(:) anticoagulation in heart disease. *BMJ*: 1999;**318**: 238–44 (website version at www.bmj.com).
Petersen P, Botsen G, Godfredsen J *et al.* Placebo-controlled, randomised trial for prevention of thromboembolic complications in chronic atrial fibrillation. The Copenhagen AFASAK Study. *Lancet* 1989;**i**: 175–9.

65　Which patients with SVT should be referred for an intracardiac electrophysiological study (EP study)? What are the success rates and risks of radiofrequency (RF) ablation?

Roy M John

The management of supraventricular tachycardia (SVT) has changed dramatically with the development of curative radiofrequency ablation (RF ablation). For most patients, the technique offers a clear alternative to long term antiarrhythmic drug therapy with its potential toxic side effects. Except for atrial fibrillation and atypical atrial flutter, most SVTs are amenable to RF ablation albeit with some variation in success rates depending on the arrhythmia mechanism.

AV nodal re-entrant tachycardia and SVTs mediated via accessory pathways are the easiest to treat with RF ablation with success rates that exceed 90%.[1] Recurrence is rare occurring in less than 10%. Focal atrial tachycardias and re-entrant atrial tachycardias resulting from prior atrial surgical scars have lower success rates of about 80%. Even for the rare but troublesome atrial tachycardia that cannot be ablated, RF ablation of the AV node with permanent cardiac pacing is effective in alleviating symptoms and can reverse any tachycardia mediated cardiomyopathy. Atrial flutter of the classical variety use a single re-entrant circuit in the right atrium and typically require an isthmus of tissue between the inferior vena cava and tricuspid valve for maintenance of the arrhythmia. RF ablation to create conduction block in this isthmus is effective in preventing recurrence of atrial flutter in 80% of patients with negligible risks. Unfortunately some patients develop atrial fibrillation because both arrhythmias share common cardiac disease processes that act as substrates for the arrhythmia mechanism. Nonetheless, fibrillation is easier to manage with drugs and combination of flutter ablation and antiarrhythmic drug therapy is often successful in maintaining sinus rhythm.

In the adult patient with the symptomatic Wolff Parkinson White syndrome, it is now generally believed that RF ablation should be the treatment of choice. Recurrent arrhythmias associated with ventricular pre-excitation are difficult to treat medically and often require the use of antiarrhythmic drugs with potent pro-arrhythmic effects or organ toxicity (e.g. flecainide, amiodarone). The risk of AV block is remote (less than 1%) unless the accessory pathway is located close to the AV node in which case the risk is higher. In infants and young children, on the other hand, it is often worth deferring RF ablation if possible because there is a chance that ventricular pre-excitation may resolve over a few years.

In contrast to the above, arrhythmias such as AV nodal re-entrant tachycardia often respond to acute or interval therapy with one of the more benign AV nodal blocking agents e.g. digoxin, beta blockers or calcium blocker. RF ablation should therefore be reserved for recurrent or troublesome arrhythmia. Situations that justify earlier RF ablative therapy include haemo-dynamic instability during episodes, intolerance of drugs, desire to avoid long term drug therapy or occupational constraints such as in airline pilots. It is also worth bearing in mind that once a patient requires more than two drugs for prophylaxis, it becomes more cost effective to proceed to RF ablation. The risk of AV block during RF ablation for AV nodal re-entrant tachycardia is between 1 and 2%,[2] and is dependent on the experience of the operator. In the younger patients, even this low rate of compli-cation can be important considering life time commitment to cardiac pacing in the event of heart block.

The risk of RF ablation is primarily that of AV block as noted above. Other risks are those related to cardiac catheterisation and include vascular damage, cardiac tamponade, myocardial infarction, cerebrovascular or pulmonary embolism and rarely damage to the valve in left sided pathways. In experienced centres, the risk of serious complications is less than 1%.

References

1 Ganz LI, Friedman PL. Medical progress: supraventricular tachycardia. *N Engl J Med* 1995;**332**: 162–73.
2 Kay GN, Epstein AE, Dailey SM *et al*. Role of radiofrequency ablation in the management of supraventricular arrhythmias: experience in 760 consecutive patients. *J Cardiovasc Electrophysiol* 1993;**4**: 371–89.

66 What drugs should I use for chemically cardioverting atrial fibrillation and when is DC cardioversion preferable?

Suzanna Hardman and Martin Cowie

Drugs are more likely to be effective when used relatively early following the onset of atrial fibrillation. However, when a clear history of recent onset atrial fibrillation has been obtained it is important to establish and treat the likely precipitants. In many instances this will allow spontaneous reversion to sinus rhythm. Important precipitants include hypoxia, dehydration, hypokalaemia, hypertension, thyrotoxicosis and coronary ischaemia. Whilst these precipitants are being treated rate control will usually be required. Short acting oral calcium channel blockers (verapamil or diltiazem) and short acting beta blockers titrated against the patients response are most effective in this setting and likely to facilitate cardioversion. Intravenous verapamil should be avoided. If a patient with new atrial fibrillation is haemodynamically compromised urgent cardioversion is required with full heparinisation. Similarly patients with fast, recent onset atrial fibrillation with broad complexes are probably best treated with early elective DC cardioversion with full heparinisation.

With the above provisos there is a role for chemical cardioversion. Amiodarone (which has class III action and mild beta blocking activity) given through a large peripheral line or centrally can be highly effective, though a rate slowing agent may also be needed. Intravenous flecainide (class I) can also be highly effective. Like other class I agents (quinidine, disopyramide and procainamide), flecainide is best avoided in patients with known or possible coronary artery disease and in conditions known to predispose to torsade de pointes. Digoxin has no role in the cardioversion of atrial fibrillation.

The highest likelihood of successful cardioversion in patients with chronic atrial fibrillation is with DC cardioversion following appropriate investigation and anticoagulation. It should be noted that cardioversion is generally safe during digoxin therapy, so long as potassium and digoxin levels are in the normal range.

Further reading

Falk RH. Proarrhythmic responses to atrial antiarrhythmic therapy. In: Falk RH, Podrid PJ, eds. *Atrial fibrillation mechanisms and management*, 2nd edition. Philadelphia: Lippincott and Raven, 1997: 371–379.

Janse MJ, Allessie MA. Experimental observations on atrial fibrillation. In: Falk RH, Podrid PJ, eds. *Atrial fibrillation mechanisms and management*. 2nd edition. Philadelphia: Lippincott and Raven, 1997: 53–73.

Nattel S, Courtemarche, Wang Z. Functional and ionic mechanisms of antiarrhythmic drugs in atrial fibrillation. In: Falk RH, Podrid PJ, eds. *Atrial fibrillation mechanisms and management*, 2nd edition. Philadelphia: Lippincott and Raven, 1997: 75–90.

67 How long should someone with atrial fibrillation be anticoagulated before DC cardioversion, and how long should this be continued afterwards?

Suzanna Hardman and Martin Cowie

For years, the rationale for a period of anticoagulation prior to cardioversion was that the anticoagulation would either stabilise or abolish any thrombus, the assumption being that thrombo-emboli associated with cardioversion occurred when effective atrial contraction was restored, dislodging pre-existing thrombus. Furthermore, it was assumed that recent onset atrial fibrillation was not associated with left atrial (LA) or left atrial appendage (LAA) thrombus and could therefore be safely cardioverted without anticoagulation. Although this has become standard clinical practice it is not evidence-based and not without hazard. With anticoagulation most thrombus appears to resolve rather than to organise. In patients with non-rheumatic atrial fibrillation most atrial thrombi will have resolved after four to six weeks of anticoagulation but persistent thrombus has been reported. Left atrial thrombus is present in a significant proportion of patients with recent onset atrial fibrillation and the associated thrombo-embolic rate is similar to that found in patients with chronic atrial fibrillation. Furthermore, cardioversion itself is associated with the development of spontaneous contrast and new thrombus and, in the absence of anticoagulation, even those patients who have had thrombus excluded using transoesophageal echocardiography have subsequently developed symptomatic thromboemboli.

For most patients a period of 4 to 6 weeks of anticoagulation and a transthoracic echocardiogram prior to cardioversion will be sufficient. Patients at high risk of thrombus (e.g. those with cardiomyopathy, mitral stenosis or previous thromboembolism) should undergo a transoesophageal study prior to cardioversion. In certain patients there may be cogent arguments for minimising the period of anticoagulation. In these patients transoesophageal echocardiography can be undertaken and provided no thrombus is identified will abolish the need for prolonged anticoagulation prior to cardioversion. However, all patients with atrial fibrillation need to be fully anticoagulated at the time of cardioversion and for a period thereafter.

The duration of post-cardioversion anticoagulation should be dictated by the likely timing of the return of normal LA/LAA function and the likelihood of maintaining sinus rhythm. If atrial fibrillation has been present for several days only, normal atrial function will usually be re-established over a similar period and intravenous heparin for a few days post-cardioversion is probably adequate. Where the duration of AF is longer or unknown a period of anticoagulation with warfarin for 1–3 months is advised (reflecting a slower time course of recovery of atrial function).

Further reading

Black IW, Fatkin D, Sagar KB *et al*. Exclusion of atrial thrombus by trans-oesoophageal echocardiography does not preclude embolism after cardioversion of atrial fibrillation. A multicenter study. *Circulation* 1994;**89**: 2509–13.

Hardman SM, Cowie M. Fortnightly review: anticoagulation in heart disease. *BMJ* 1999;**318**: 238–44 (website version at www.bmj.com).

Stoddard MF, Dawkins PR, Prince CR *et al*. Left atrial appendage thrombus is not uncommon in patients with acute atrial fibrillation and a recent embolic event; a transoesophageal echocardiographic study. *J Am Coll Cardiol* 1995;**25**: 452–9.

68 What factors determine the chances of successful elective cardioversion from atrial fibrillation?

Suzanna Hardman and Martin Cowie

Elective cardioversion should only be undertaken when the precipitant (e.g. hypoxia, ischaemia, thyrotoxicosis, hypokalaemia and hypoglycaemia) has been treated and the patient is metabolically stable. With this proviso, the success of cardioversion depends not so much on the ability to *restore* sinus rhythm (success rates of 70–90% are usual), but rather on the capacity to *sustain* sinus rhythm.

Cardioversion of unselected patients will result in consistently high rates of relapse: at one year 40 to 80% of patients will have reverted to atrial fibrillation. Early cardioversion, particularly in those patients in whom a clear trigger of atrial fibrillation has been effectively treated and in whom there is little or no evidence of concomitant cardiac disease, is associated with the best long term outcome. This may reflect the finding (well described in animal models) that sustained atrial fibrillation modifies atrial electro-physiology so that, with time, there is a predisposition to continued and recurrent AF. If early cardioversion is not feasible, then the extent of underlying cardiac disease may be a more important determinant of long term outcome than the duration of AF.

The presence of severe structural cardiac disease is associated with a high relapse rate and sometimes an inability to achieve cardioversion, e.g. severe ventricular dysfunction, markedly enlarged atria and valvular disease.

Certain categories of patients justify specific mention:

- Obese patients may be especially resistant to cardioversion from the external route but not necessarily using electrodes positioned within the heart.
- A proportion of patients with paroxysmal atrial fibrillation will eventually develop chronic atrial fibrillation: for many this provides a paradoxical reprieve from their symptoms. If cardioverted their propensity to atrial fibrillation remains and they are likely to relapse.
- The prognosis of patients with structurally normal hearts who develop atrial fibrillation as a result of thyrotoxicosis is

excellent: once the thyrotoxicosis has been treated a high proportion revert to sinus rhythm and the remainder are sensitive to cardioversion with a relatively low relapse.

Further reading

Hardman SMC. Ventricular function in atrial fibrillation. In: Falk RH, Podrid PJ, eds. *Atrial fibrillation mechanisms and management*, 2nd edition. Philadelphia: Lippincott and Raven, 1997: 91–108.

Nakazawa H, Lythall DA, Noh J *et al*. Is there a place for the late cardioversion of atrial fibrillation? A long-term follow-up study of patients with post-thyrotoxic atrial fibrillation. *Eur Heart J*; **21**: 327–333.

Van Gelder IC, Crijns HJ, Van Gilst WH *et al*. Prediction of uneventful cardioversion and maintenance of sinus rhythm from direct current electrical cardioversion of chronic atrial fibrillation and flutter. *Am J Cardiol* 1991;**68**: 41–6.

Wijffels MCEF, Kirchhof CJHJ, Dorland R *et al*. Atrial fibrillation begets atrial fibrillation. A study in awake chronically instrumented goats. *Circulation* 1995;**92**: 1954–68.

69 What are the risks of elective DC cardioversion from atrial fibrillation?

Suzanna Hardman and Martin Cowie

There are relatively few recent published data on the risks of elective DC cardioversion. The risks include those relating to an, albeit brief, general anaesthetic which will reflect the overall health of the patient, and those relating to the application of synchronised direct current shock. The latter include the development of bradyarrhythmias (more likely in the presence of heavy beta blockade and especially where there is concomitant use of calcium channel antagonists) and tachyarrhythmias (more likely in the presence of deranged biochemistry including low serum K^+ or Mg^{++}, and high levels of serum digoxin). These dysrhythmias may necessitate emergency pacing or further cardioversion and full resuscitation. Elective cardioversion of adequately assessed patients should only be undertaken by appropriately trained staff in an area where full resuscitation facilities are available. Following cardioversion high quality nursing care and ECG monitoring will be required until the patient has recovered from the anaesthetic and is clinically stable. Failure to observe these guidelines will likely result in higher complication rates which on occasion includes death.

The other major complication of DC cardioversion is thromboembolism which can be debilitating and is sometimes fatal. There have been no randomised trials of anticoagulation but there is convincing circumstantial evidence that anti-coagulation reduces the risk of cardioversion-related thrombo-embolism from figures in the order of 7% to less than 1%: anticoagulation does not appear to abolish the risk and this should be made explicit when informed consent is obtained from a patient. Patients with recent onset AF are not devoid of the risks of cardioversion-related thromboembolism and also require anticoagulation.

Further reading
Bjerkelund CJ, Orning OM. The efficacy of anticoagulant therapy in preventing embolism related to DC electrical cardioversion of atrial fibrillation. *Am J Cardiol* 1969;**23**: 208–16.

Schnittger I. Value of transoesophageal echocardiography before DC cardioversion in patients with atrial fibrillation: assessment of embolic risk. *Br Heart J* 1995;**73**: 306–9.

Yurchack PM, for Task Force Members: Williams SV, Achford JL, Reynolds WA *et al*. AHA/ACC/ACP Task Force statement. Clinical competence in elective direct current (DC) cardioversion. *Circulation* 1993;**88**: 342–5.

70 Are patients with atrial flutter at risk of embolisation when cardioverted? Do they need anticoagulation to cover the procedure?

Suzanna Hardman and Martin Cowie

Although common clinical practice and guidelines do not advocate routine anticoagulation of patients with atrial flutter undergoing cardioversion, there are no data to support this practice. Rather, recent studies suggest the prevalence of intra-atrial thrombus in unselected patients with atrial flutter is significant and of the order of 30–35% (compared with 3% prevalence in a control population in sinus rhythm). The atrial standstill (or stunning) that has been described post-cardioversion of atrial fibrillation and is thought to be a factor in the associated thromboembolic risk has also now been described immediately post-cardioversion of patients with atrial flutter. Although some authors argue that the stunning post-cardioversion of atrial flutter is "attenuated" compared with the response in atrial fibrillation, the thromboembolic rate associated with cardioversion of atrial flutter in the absence of anticoagulation argues against this. Indeed, the thromboembolic rate appears to be comparable with the early experience of cardioverting atrial fibrillation. Furthermore, atrial flutter is an intrinsically unstable rhythm which may degenerate into atrial fibrillation and certain patients alternate between atrial fibrillation and atrial flutter.

Like atrial fibrillation, atrial flutter may be the first manifestation of underlying heart disease and it is likely, though not yet proven, that the thromboembolic risks associated with both chronic atrial flutter and with cardioversion of atrial flutter vary with the extent of underlying cardiovascular pathology. Although existing data are limited, on current evidence we advise that patients with atrial flutter should be anticoagulated prior to, during and post-cardioversion, in the same way as patients with atrial fibrillation.

Further reading

Bikkina M, Alpert MA, Madhuri M *et al*. Prevalence of intra-atrial thrombus in patients with atrial flutter. *Am J Cardiol* 1995;**76**;186–9.
Irani WN, Grayburn PA, Afrii I. Prevalence of thrombus, spontaneous echo contrast, and atrial stunning in patients undergoing cardioversion

of atrial flutter. A prospective study using transoesophageal echocardiography. *Circulation* 1997;**95**: 962–6.

Jordaens L, Missault L, Germonpre E *et al.* Delayed restoration of atrial function after cardioversion of atrial flutter by pacing or electrical cardioversion. *Am J Cardiol* 1993;**71**: 63–6.

Mehta D, Baruch L. Thromboembolism following cardioversion of common atrial flutter. Risk factors and limitations of transoesophageal echocardiography. *Chest* 1996;**110**: 1001–3.

71 How do I assess the risk of CVA or TIA in a patient with chronic atrial fibrillation and in a patient with paroxysmal atrial fibrillation?

Suzanna Hardman and Martin Cowie

Age is an important determinant of the risk of thrombo-embolism, and hence of transient ischaemic attack (TIA) and of cerebrovascular accident (CVA) in patients with atrial fibrillation. If the patient is aged less than 60 years, and has no evidence of other cardiac disease (such as coronary artery disease, valve disease or heart failure) the risk of thrombo-embolism is low (of the order of 0.5% per year). This risk is lower than the risk of a serious bleed if the patient is anticoagulated with warfarin (1.3% per year or higher depending on the quality of anticoagulation control). If the patient is older than the 60 years, or has evidence of other cardiovascular disease, the risk of thromboembolism increases.

In the Stroke Prevention in Atrial Fibrillation Study clinical features indicating a higher risk of thromboembolism were: age over 60 years; history of congestive heart failure within the previous 3 months; hypertension (treated or untreated); and previous thromboembolism. The more of these features present in a patient the higher the risk of thromboembolism. A large left atrium (>2.5cm diameter/m² body surface area) or global left ventricular systolic dysfunction on transthoracic echo-cardiography also identifies patients at a higher risk of thrombo-embolism. Such abnormalities may not be suspected clinically and wherever possible echocardiography should be performed in patients with AF in order to determine more precisely the risk of thromboembolism.

Paroxysmal (as opposed to chronic) atrial fibrillation covers a wide spectrum of disease severity with the duration and frequency of attacks varying markedly between and within patients. Although the clinical trials of anticoagulation in patients with atrial fibrillation were inconsistent in including patients with paroxysmal atrial fibrillation, there was no evidence that such patients had a lower risk of thromboembolism than those with chronic atrial fibrillation. It is likely that as the episodes become more frequent and of longer duration that the risk approaches those in patients with chronic atrial fibrillation.

Further reading

Hardman SMC, Cowie M. Fortnightly review: anticoagulation in heart disease. *BMJ* 1999;**318**: 238–244 (website version at www.bmj.com.)

The Stroke Prevention in Atrial Fibrillation Investigators. Predictors of thromboembolism in atrial fibrillation I. Clinical features of thrombo-embolism in atrial fibrillation. *Ann Intern Med* 1992;**116**: 1–5.

The Stroke Prevention in Atrial Fibrillation Investigators. Predictors of thromboembolism in atrial fibrillation II. Echocardiographic features of patients at risk. *Ann Intern Med* 1992;**116**: 6–12.

72 How sensitive are transthoracic and transoesophageal echocardiography for the detection of thrombus in the left atrium?

Suzanna Hardman and Martin Cowie

The ability of echocardiography to detect left atrial clot is determined by the sophistication of the equipment, the ease with which the left atrium and left atrial appendage can be scanned and the skill and experience of the operator. Historically, at best, the sensitivity of two dimensional transthoracic echocardiography for detecting left atrial thrombus has been of the order of 40–65%, with the left atrial appendage visualised in under 20% of patients even in experienced hands. This compared with a reported sensitivity of 75–95% for visualising left ventricular thrombi from the transthoracic approach. More recent data, from a tertiary referral centre using the new generation transthoracic echocardiography, suggest the left atrial appendage can be adequately imaged in 75% of patients and that within this group 91% of thrombi identified by transoesophageal echocardiography will also be visualised from the transthoracic approach. Although encouraging, the extent to which these figures can be reproduced using similar equipment by the generality of units remains to be established.

Available data for the sensitivity of transoesophageal echocardiography in detecting left atrial and left atrial appendage thrombus consistently report a high positive predictive value. The largest series of 231 patients identified thrombus ranging from 3 to 80mm in 14 patients: compared with findings at surgery this produced a sensitivity of 100%. But these findings need to be interpreted with considerable caution and are unlikely to be applicable to all users of the technique. The study was carried out in a tertiary referral centre with a particular interest and long-standing investment in the technique and the nine observers involved in reporting the data all had extensive experience. Nonetheless, transoesophageal echocardiography is undoubtedly the investigation of choice for imaging the left atrium and left atrial appendage.

Further reading

Aschenberg W, Schiuter M, Kremer P *et al*. Transoesophageal two-dimensional echocardiography for the detection of left atrial appendage thrombus. *J Am Coll Cardiol* 1986;**7**: 163–6.

Manning WJ, Weintraub RM, Waksmonski CA *et al*. Accuracy of trans-oesophageal echocardiography for identifying left atrial thrombi. A prospective intraoperative study. *Ann Intern Med* 1995;**123**: 817–22.

Omran H, Jung W, Rabahieh R *et al*. Imaging of thrombi and assessment of left atrial appendage function: a prospective study comparing trans-thoracic and transoesophageal echocardiography. *Heart* 1999;**81**: 192–8.

Schweizer P, Bardos P, Erbel R *et al*. Detection of left atrial thrombi by echocardiography. *Br Heart J* 1981;**45**: 148–56.

73 What are the roles of transthoracic and transoesophageal echocardiography in patients with a TIA or stroke?

Diana Holdright

Approximately 80% of strokes are ischaemic in origin, of which 20–40% have a cardiac basis. TIAs have a cardiac cause in ~15% of cases. Common cardiac abnormalities associated with neuro-logical events include atrial fibrillation, mitral valve disease, left atrial enlargement, left ventricular dilatation, prosthetic valve abnormalities and endocarditis. Clinical examination and simple tests (CXR and ECG) should indicate cardiac abnormality in these situations. The aim of echocardiography is to confirm the presence of important predisposing cardiac abnormalities and in younger patients, typically <50 years, to look for rare cardiac causes that might not be detected by other means. This latter group includes atrial septal aneurysm and patent foramen ovale (PFO) which, although somewhat controversial, are associated with an increased risk of stroke in patients without other detectable abnormalities.

Consequently, echocardiography is particularly useful in patients at both ends of the age scale. Older patients are more likely to have cardiac abnormalities that could give rise to stroke/TIA and young patients frequently have apparently normal hearts, but echocardiography (especially trans-oesophageal) may indicate the presence of an atrial septal aneurysm or PFO. The pick-up rate of transthoracic echocardiog-raphy is extremely low in patients with a normal clinical exami-nation, CXR and ECG, making it a poor screening test. Conversely, the yield in patients with clinical abnormalities or an abnormal ECG/CXR is high and may give useful information for risk strat-ification beyond simply confirming a clinical diagnosis, for example left atrial size and the presence of spontaneous contrast.

Transoesophageal echocardiography should be reserved for "younger" patients (empirically <50 years) with unexplained stroke/TIA, for patients in whom the transthoracic study is unclear, and for older patients with repeated unexplained stroke/TIA. Transoesophageal echocardiography is particularly useful for looking at the left atrium, atrial septum, left atrial appendage, mitral valve and thoracic aorta, abnormalities of which may give rise to stroke/TIA. There is a tendency to over-report more subtle abnormalities (e.g. slight mitral valve prolapse) that may not be clinically relevant.

Further reading

Nighoghossian N, Perinetti M, Barthelet M *et al.* Potential cardioembolic sources of stroke in patients less than 60 years of age. *Eur Heart J* 1996;**17**: 590–4.

Pearson AC, Labovitz AJ, Tatineni S *et al.* Superiority of trans-oesophageal echocardiography in detecting cardiac source of embolism in patients with cerebral ischaemia of uncertain aetiology. *J Am Coll Cardiol* 1991;**17**: 66–72.

74 Which patient with a patent foramen ovale should be referred for closure?

Diana Holdright

A patent foramen ovale (PFO) occurs in approximately one quarter of the population. It is a vestige of the fetal circulation, with an orifice varying in size from 1 to 19mm, allowing right-to-left or bidirectional shunting at atrial level and the potential for paradoxical embolism. The development of better imaging techniques (e.g. transoesophageal echocardiography, contrast agents) and the fact that 35% of ischaemic strokes remain unexplained has generated interest in the potential for paradoxical thromboembolism through a PFO.

Studies of patients with cryptogenic stroke give a higher incidence of PFO (up to 56%)[1] than in a control population, suggesting, but not proving, causality. Stroke due to paradoxical embolism involves the passage of material across a PFO, at a time when right atrial pressure exceeds left atrial pressure, to the brain. In one study the incidence of venous thrombosis as the sole risk factor for presumed embolic stroke in patients with PFOs was 9.5% and was clinically silent in 80% of patients,[2] adding support to the concept of paradoxical embolism. The detection of venous thrombosis is not without difficulty and venous thrombi may resolve with time, such that a negative study does not exclude prior thrombosis. There is evidence that PFOs allow right-to-left shunting under normal physiological conditions, during coughing, straining and similar manoeuvres and especially in patients with raised right heart pressures and tricuspid regurgitation.

There are no completed prospective trials comparing aspirin, warfarin and percutaneous closure to guide management of patients with an ischaemic stroke presumed to be cardioembolic in origin. Opinion is divided in the case of a single ischaemic lesion on MR imaging and an isolated PFO – there is no evidence in favour of any particular strategy. Aspirin therapy is an uncomplicated option, and easier and safer than life-long warfarin. If there is evidence of more than one ischaemic lesion, no indication for warfarin (e.g. a procoagulant state), preferably a history of a Valsalva manoeuvre or equivalent immediately preceding the stroke and no alternative cause for the stroke then I would consider percutaneous closure, which has rapidly developed as a highly effective and technically straightforward procedure for closure of PFOs and many atrial septal defects.

References

1 Cabanes L, Mas JL, Cohen A *et al.* Atrial septal aneurysm and patent foramen ovale as risk factors for cryptogenic stroke in patients less than 55 years of age. *Stroke* 1993;**24**: 1865–73.

2 Lethen H, Flachskampf FA, Schneider R *et al.* Frequency of deep vein thrombosis in patients with patent foramen ovale and ischemic stroke or transient ischemic attack. *Am J Cardiol* 1997;**80**: 1066–9.

75 How should I investigate the patient with collapse? Who should have a tilt test, and what do I do if it is positive?

RA Kenny and Diarmuid O'Shea

Investigation of a patient with collapse

The history from the older patient may be less reliable, however a careful history often allows syncopal episodes to be classified into broad diagnostic categories (Table 75.1). Elderly patients may have amnesia for their collapse. A witness history, available in only 40–60% of cases, can thus be invaluable. Witnessed features of prodrome (i.e. pallor, sweating, loss of consciousness or fitting) and clinical characteristics after the event can all help in building a diagnostic picture. Physical examination should include an assessment of blood pressure in the supine and erect position, a cardiovascular examination to look for the presence or absence of structural heart disease (including aortic stenosis, mitral stenosis, outflow tract obstruction, atrial myxoma or impaired left ventricular function) and auscultation for carotid bruits. The 12-lead electrocardiogram (ECG) remains an important tool in the diagnosis of arrhythmic syncope. Up to 11% of syncopal patients have a diagnosis assigned from their ECG. More importantly those with a normal 12-lead ECG (no QRS or rhythm distur-bance) have a low likelihood of arrhythmia as a cause of their syncope and are at low risk of sudden death. Thus the history and physical examination can guide you as to the more appropriate diagnostic tests for the individual patient and would include the following:

- ECG
- 24 hour ECG
- 24 hour BP
- Carotid sinus massage – supine and erect (only if negative supine)
- External loop recorder
- Electrophysiological studies
- Head up tilt test
- CT head and EEG if appropriate
- Implantable loop recorder

Table 75.1 Clinical features suggestive of a specific cause of syncope

Diagnostic consideration	Symptom or finding
Neurally mediated	
Carotid sinus syncope	Syncope with head rotation
Vasovagal syncope	After pain, unpleasant sight or sound
	Prolonged standing
	Athlete after exertion
Situational	Micturition, cough, swallow, defecation
Orthostatic	On standing
Post-prandial	After meals
Cardiogenic	
Structural heart disease – aortic and mitral stenosis	Syncope on exertion
Ischaemic heart disease	
Non-cardiovascular	
Seizures	Witness fitting
Cerebrovascular disease	Associated with vertigo, dysarthria, diplopia or other motor and sensory symptoms of brain stem ischaemia
Subclavian steal	Syncope with arm exercise

Modified from Kenny RA ed., *Syncope in the older patient*. Chapman and Hall Medical 1996.

Who should have a tilt test?

Kenny *et al* in 1986 were the first to demonstrate the value of head up tilt testing in the diagnosis of unexplained syncope.[1] There is a broad group of hypotensive syndromes and conditions where head up tilt testing should be considered – patients with recurrent syncope or presyncope and high risk patients with a history of a single syncopal episode (serious injury during episode, driving) where no other cause for symptoms is suggested by initial history, examination or cardiovascular and neurological investigations. Tilt table testing may also be of use in the assessment of elderly patients with recurrent unexplained falls and in the differential diagnosis of convulsive syncope, orthostatic hypotension, postural tachycardia syndrome, psychogenic and hyperventilation syncope and carotid sinus hypersensitivity.

What do you do if you make a diagnosis of vasovagal syncope on history and head up tilt test?

As a result of the complexity of the aetiology of vasovagal syncope and the lack of a single well evaluated therapeutic intervention there are many treatments available. These have recently been reviewed,[2] and the following algorithm for management of vasovagal syncope suggested (Algorithm 75.1).

References
1 Kenny RA, Ingram A, Bayliss J *et al*. Head-up tilt: a useful test for investigating unexplained syncope. *Lancet* 1986;**i**: 1352–4.
2 Parry SW, Kenny RA. The management of vasovagal syncope. *Q J Med* 1999;**92**: 697–705.

Further reading
Kenny RA, O'Shea D, Parry SW. The Newcastle protocols for head-up tilt table testing in the diagnosis of vasovagal syncope and related disorders. *Heart* 2000;**83**: 564–9.

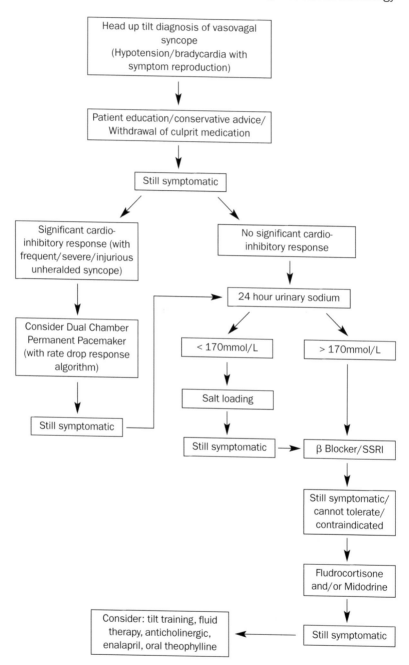

Algorithm 75.1 Management of vasovagal syncope

76 What are the chances of a 24 hour tape detecting the causes for collapse in a patient? What other alternative monitoring devices are now available?

RA Kenny and Diarmuid O'Shea

Syncope is a common medical problem accounting for up to 6% of emergency medical admissions. In older patients presenting to casualty this may be as high as 20% when evaluated with a full cardiovascular work up. The annual recurrence rate is as high as 30%.[1] Syncope due to cardiac causes is associated with a high mortality (>50% at 5 years) compared with 30% at 5 years in patients with syncope due to non-cardiac syncope and 24% in those with unexplained syncope.[2] However, in the elderly, even "benign" syncope can result in significant morbidity and mortality due to trauma, anxiety or depression, which may lead to major changes in lifestyle or financial difficulties.[3]

Syncope is often unpredictable in onset, intermittent and has a high rate of spontaneous remission making it a difficult diagnostic challenge. Thus even after a thorough work up, the cause of syncope may remain unexplained in up to 40% of cases.[4] Prolonged ambulatory monitoring is often used as a first line investigation. Documentation of significant arrhythmias or syncope during monitoring is rare. At best, symptoms correlating with arrhythmias occur in 4% of patients, asymptomatic arrhythmias occur in up to 13%, and symptoms without arrhythmias occur in up to a further 17%.[5-7] Prolonged monitoring may result in a slight increase in diagnostic yield from 15% with 24 hours of monitoring to 29% at 72 hours.[8]

Patient activated external loop recorders have a higher diagnostic yield but do not yield a symptom-rhythm correlation in over 66% of patients, either because of device malfunction, patient non-compliance or an inability to activate the recorder.[9,10] In addition such devices are only useful in patients with relatively frequent symptoms. In a follow up by Kapoor *et al*,[11] only 5% of patients reported recurrent symptoms at 1 month, 11% at 3 months and 16% at 6 months. Thus this type of monitoring is likely to be useful only in a small subgroup of patients with frequent recurrence in whom initial evaluation is negative and arrhythmias are not diagnosed by other means, such as 24 hour ECG or electrophysiology studies.

The diagnostic yield from cardiac electrophysiology ranges from 14–70%. This variability is primarily dependent on the characteristics of patients studied, in particular the absence or presence of co-morbid cardiovascular disease.[12] Thus despite the use of investigations such as head up tilt testing, ambulatory cardiac monitoring, external loop recorders and electrophysiological testing, the underlying cause of syncope remains unexplained and continues to pose a diagnostic problem.

The implantable loop recorder (ILR) is a new diagnostic tool to add to the strategies for investigation of unexplained syncope.[12] It permits long term cardiac monitoring to capture the ECG during a spontaneous episode in patients without recurrence in a reasonable time frame. It should be considered in those who have already completed the above outlined investigations that have proved negative, and in those in whom the external loop recorder has not yielded a diagnosis in one month. The ILR is implanted under local anaesthetic via a small incision usually in the left pectoral region. It has the ability to "freeze" the current and preceding rhythm for up to 40 minutes after a spontaneous event and thus allows the determination of the cause of syncope in most patients in whom symptoms are due to an arrhythmia. The activation device, used by the patient, family member or friend freezes and stores the loop during and after a spontaneous syncopal episode. This is retrievable at a later stage using a standard pacemaker programmer. The ILR specifically monitors heart rate changes. Hypotensive syndromes including vasovagal syncope, orthostatic hypotension, post-prandial hypotension and vasodepressor carotid sinus hypersensivity may also cause syncope. An ability to record blood pressure variation in addition to heart rate changes during symptoms would be a very helpful and exciting addition to the investigation of people with syncope.

References

1 Brady PA, Shen WK. Syncope evaluation in the elderly. *Am J Geriatr Cardiol* 1999;**8**: 115–24.
2 Kapoor W. Syncope in older persons. *J Am Geriatr Soc* 1994;**42**: 426–36.
3 Lipsitz L. Syncope in the elderly. *Ann Intern Med* 1983;**99**: 92–105.
4 Kapoor W. Diagnostic evaluation of syncope. *Am J Med* 1991;**90**: 91–106.
5 Gibson TC, Heitzman MK. Diagnostic efficacy of 24 hour electrocardiographic monitoring for syncope. *Am J Cardiol* 1984;**53**: 1013–17.
6 Clark PI, Glasser SO, Spoto E. Arrhythmias detected by ambulatory monitoring; lack of correlation with symptoms of dizziness and syncope. *Chest* 1990;**77**: 722–5.

7 DiMarco P, Philbrick JT. Use of ambulatory electrocardiographic (Holter) monitoring. *Ann Intern Med* 1990;**113**: 53–68.

8 Bass EB, Curtiss EI, Arena VC. The duration of holter monitoring in patients with syncope: is 24 hours enough? *Arch Intern Med* 1990;**150**: 1073–8.

9 Linzer M, Pritchett ELC, Pontiueu M *et al.* Incremental diagnostic yield of loop electrocardiographic recorders in unexplained syncope. *Am J Cardiol* 1990;**66**: 214–19.

10 Brown AD, Dawkins RD, Davies JG. Detection of arrhythmias; use of patient-activated ambulatory electrocardiogram device with a solid state memory loop. *Br Heart J* 1989;**58**: 251–3.

11 Kapoor W, Peterson J, Wieand H *et al.* Diagnostic and prognostic implications of recurrences in patients with syncope. *Am J Med* 1987;**83**: 700–8.

12 Kenny RA, Krahn AD. Implantable loop recorder: evaluation of unexplained syncope. *Heart* 1999;**81**: 431–3.

77 Should the patient with trifascicular disease be routinely paced? If not, why not?

Simon Sporton

Normal activation of the ventricles below the bundle of His occurs by way of three "fascicles" – the right bundle branch and the anterosuperior and posteroinferior divisions of the left bundle branch. Conduction block in two of the three fascicles is bifascicular block. Additional prolongation of the PR interval results in "trifascicular block" implying abnormal conduction through or above the remaining fascicle. The concern is that conduction will fail in the remaining fascicle, i.e. complete heart block will develop with a slow and unreliable ventricular escape rhythm. Potential consequences include syncope and death.

There have been no randomised trials of pacing vs no pacing in patients with chronic bi- or trifascicular block. Clinicians must therefore be guided by knowledge of the natural history of the condition without pacing, and expert consensus guidelines.

The largest prospective study of patients with bi- and trifascicular block followed 554 asymptomatic patients for a mean of 42 months. The five year mortality from an event that may conceivably have been a bradyarrhythmia was just 6%, a figure that must inevitably include some non-bradyarrhythmic deaths. The five year incidence of complete heart block was also low at 5%. A prolonged PR interval was associated with a higher incidence of potentially bradyarrhythmic deaths but not with the development of complete heart block. An important finding of this study was a five year all cause mortality of 35% reflecting the high incidence of underlying coronary heart disease and congestive cardiac failure.

The available evidence would suggest that asymptomatic patients with trifascicular block should not be paced routinely. A history of syncope should prompt thorough investigation for both brady- and tachyarrhythmic causes. If intermittent second or third degree block is documented permanent pacing is indicated. If tachyarrhythmias are implicated then therapy is likely to include antiarrhythmic drugs, which may exacerbate AV block and prophylactic permanent pacing would seem wise. Bi- and trifascicular block are associated with a high incidence of underlying coronary heart disease and heart failure. Attention should therefore be directed towards the detection of these conditions and the use of therapies known to improve their prognosis.

Further reading

Gregoratos G, Cheitlin MD, Conill A *et al.* ACC/AHA guidelines for implantation of cardiac pacemakers and antiarrhythmia devices. *J Am Coll Cardiol* 1998;**31**: 1175–209.

McAnulty JH, Rahimtoola SH, Murphy E *et al.* Natural history of "high-risk" bundle-branch block. *N Engl J Med* 1982;**307**: 137–43.

78 Who should have VVI pacemakers and who should have dual chamber pacemakers? What are the risks of pacemaker insertion?

Alistair Slade

Many pacing enthusiasts argue that there are very few indications for VVI pacing, perhaps confining its role to the very elderly with established atrial fibrillation and documented pauses. Dual chamber pacing (or more accurately physiological pacing which may include single chamber atrial devices) is the preferred mode in most common indications for pacemaker implantation.

The British Pacing group published its recommendations in 1991.[1] These have led to widespread if gradual change in British pacing practice. Physiological pacemakers can be recommended in sinus node disease on the basis of many retrospective studies and one prospective study.[2] Ongoing prospective studies will clarify the true role of physiological pacing in the elderly with AV conduction disease. The British guidelines are similar to those in the United States. A more comprehensive guide to pacemaker implantation is given by the ACC/AHA joint guidelines which supply the level of evidence for each recommendation and a comprehensive reference list.[3]

Pacemaker implantation is a remarkably safe procedure. Mortality is minimal and occurs due to unrecognised pneumothorax, pericardial tamponade or great vessel trauma. Complications at implant are those of subclavian puncture, particularly pneumothorax, although these can be avoided if the cephalic approach is used. There is some long term evidence that the cephalic approach may avoid chronic lead failure in polyurethane leads due to subclavian crush injury. Haematoma requiring re-operation should occur in less than 1%. Infection leading to explant similarly occurs in approximately 1%. Acute lead displacement should be less than 1% for ventricular leads and 1–2% for atrial leads.

References

1 Clark M, Sutton R, Ward DE *et al*. Recommendations for pacemaker prescription for symptomatic bradycardia. Report of a working party of the British Pacing and Electrophysiology Group. *Br Heart J* 1991;**66**: 185–91.

2 Andersen HR, Thuesen L, Bagger JP *et al.* Prospective randomised trial of atrial versus ventricular pacing in sick-sinus syndrome. *Lancet* 1994;**344**: 1523–8.

3 Gregoratos G, Cheitlin MD, Conill A *et al.* ACC/AHA guidelines for implantation of cardiac pacemakers and antiarrhythmia devices. *J Am Coll Cardiol* 1998;**31**: 1175–209.

79 Can a patient with a pacemaker touch an electric fence? ...have an MRI scan? ...go through airport metal detectors? ...use a mobile phone?

Alistair Slade

Pacemakers have increasingly sophisticated circuitry to prevent damage or interference from external magnetic interference.

Electric fences

Nobody should touch an electric fence but should electric shock occur it would be wise to have the system checked by formal interrogation in case electrical mode reversion has occurred.

Magnetic Resonance Imaging (MRI)

MRI poses potential problems for the pacemaker patient. Significant artefact would be obtained in regions close to an implanted pacemaker but more importantly the powerful magnetic fields might interfere with the device. Initial blanket denial of MRI imaging to the pacemaker patient has been tempered by small studies showing device safety under carefully controlled conditions. Extreme caution should be advised and expert opinion sought prior to planned MRI investigation.

Airport metal detectors

Airport metal detectors have the potential to interfere with pacing systems. Patients should produce their pacemaker registration cards to bypass busy security queues.

Mobile phones

Mobile phones have been extensively investigated in terms of interaction with implanted devices. *Analogue phones* do not interact with implanted devices but more modern *digital devices* have the potential to interfere with pacing systems when utilised within a field of 10–15 cm. Pacemaker patients with mobile phones are therefore advised to carry mobile telephones on the opposite side of the body from the site of the device implant and should hold the device to the opposite ear.

Further reading

Gimbel JR, Johnson D, Levine PA *et al*. Safe performance of magnetic resonance imaging on five patients with permanent cardiac pacemakers. *Pacing Clin Electrophysiol* 1996;**19**: 913–19.

Hayes DL, Wang PJ, Reynolds DW *et al*. Interference with cardiac pacemakers by cellular telephones. *N Engl J Med* 1997;**336**: 1473–9.

80 What do I do if a patient has a pacemaker and needs cardioversion?

Alistair Slade

Patients with pacemakers often require cardioversion, particularly with the increasing use of pacing techniques in the management of paroxysmal atrial fibrillation.

Some centres reprogramme or inactivate pacemakers prior to cardioversion. The decision regarding this should be made on an individual basis, depending on the type of pacemaker, reason for implant, and pacing-dependency.

Patients needing cardioversion should have the paddles applied in a manner such that the electrical field is remote from the pacemaker electrical field. In practise the standard apex—sternum approach is safe with a pacemaker in the left shoulder region, although anteroposterior paddle positioning can be utilised. The lowest energy possible should be administered, and the pacemaker should be checked formally after the procedure as occasionally the pacemaker may change mode as a consequence of cardioversion. Efforts should be made to ensure that, during synchronised shock, the defibrillator is recognising the ventricular, and not atrial, pacing spike.

Modern systems have increasingly effective protection from external interference.

81 What do I do about non-sustained ventricular tachycardia on a 24 hour tape?

Simon Sporton

The term non-sustained ventricular tachycardia (VT) is used conventionally to describe salvos lasting a minimum of four consecutive ventricular beats and a maximum of 30 seconds in the absence of intervention. The concerns are that the non-sustained VT may itself cause symptoms of palpitation, presyncope or syncope and that the arrhythmia may persist or degenerate into ventricular fibrillation. The finding of non-sustained VT on a 24 hour tape should prompt the following questions: firstly, is there evidence of underlying heart disease; secondly, what is the morphology of the VT; thirdly, what are the patient's symptoms?

An arrhythmia is usually although not invariably a sign of underlying heart disease. This is an important consideration because treatment of the underlying condition, where possible, is likely to be more effective than antiarrhythmic drug therapy both in terms of preventing the arrhythmia and improving prognosis. Conversely, if treatable underlying heart disease remains untreated then antiarrhythmic drug therapy is unlikely to be successful.

The morphology of the VT may help to guide management: for example if torsade de pointes is observed then management will focus on adjustment of drug regimes and treatment of electrolyte deficiencies and bradycardia. The finding of monomorphic VT might suggest the presence of a re-entrant circuit or automatic focus that may be amenable to mapping and modification or ablation. Non-torsade polymorphic VT is typically seen in the context of heart failure and is seldom reliably induced by electrophysiological study or amenable to radiofrequency ablation.

There is little evidence that antiarrhythmic drug therapy alters prognosis in patients with non-sustained VT. This may reflect a lack of efficacy and/or toxicity of currently available antiarrhythmic agents. Another explanation is that non-sustained VT is frequently a marker of underlying heart disease, which itself determines prognosis. There is evidence that implantable cardioverter-defibrillators (ICDs) may improve the prognosis of patients with poor left ventricular function, *asymptomatic* non-sustained VT and inducible, non-suppressible VT following myocardial infarction. However, many important questions remain about the prophylactic implantation of ICDs in such patients. The decision to implant is easier if there is a history of presyncope or syncope.

Further reading

Buxton AE, Marchlinski FE, Waxman HL *et al.* Prognostic factors in nonsustained ventricular tachycardia. *Am J Cardiol* 1984;**53**: 1275–9.

Campbell RWF. Ventricular ectopic beats and nonsustained ventricular tachycardia. *Lancet* 1993;**341**: 1454–8.

Moss AJ, Hall WJ, Cannom DS *et al.* Improved survival with an implanted defibrillator in patients with coronary artery disease at high risk for ventricular arrhythmia. *N Engl J Med* 1996;**335**: 1933–40.

82 How do I treat torsade de pointes at a cardiac arrest?

Simon Sporton

Consideration of the electrophysiological disturbances pre-disposing to the development of torsade de pointes provides a logical approach to management. Experimental and clinical evidence impli-cates abnormal prolongation of cardiac action potential as a critical factor. Under these conditions early after-depolarisations may occur and lead to repetitive discharges ("triggered activity").

Drugs that prolong cardiac action potential and are associated with torsade include antiarrhythmic agents of class Ia and III, tricyclic antidepressants, phenothiazines, macrolide antibiotics, certain antihistamines and cisapride. Hypokalaemia and hypo-magnesaemia are well recognised causes of torsade although the evidence for hypocalcaemia is less convincing. Bradycardia – either sinus or due to atrioventricular block – is an important contributory factor.

In the setting of cardiac arrest torsade should be managed with synchronised DC cardioversion which is almost always successful in restoring sinus rhythm. However, additional measures will be necessary to prevent recurrence. These measures are aimed at shortening cardiac action potential duration. The heart rate should be increased. Atropine has the advantage of rapid availability and ease of administration. Where the brady-cardia is due to atrioventricular block atropine is unlikely to increase the ventricular rate. Transvenous ventricular pacing should be established rapidly although it is almost certainly wise to stabilise the patient first with an isoprenaline infusion (at a rate of 1-10micrograms/min, titrated against the heart rate) or external cardiac pacing. There is experimental and clinical evidence to support the use of intravenous magnesium in the acute treatment of torsade. A dose of 8mmol (administered over 10-15 minutes) has been shown to abolish torsade in the majority of patients although a second dose may be necessary. There is no evidence to support the use of either intravenous potassium or calcium. The serum concentration of these electrolytes is frequently disturbed as a result of cardiac arrest *per se* and a reasonable strategy would be to obtain a formal laboratory meas-urement after a period of haemodynamic stability and to correct as necessary. Ventricular pacing should be maintained and the ECG monitored while the factors predisposing to the development of torsade are considered and corrected. There is no role for conventional antiarrhythmic drugs in the management of torsade de pointes: on the contrary many antiarrhythmics may aggravate the situation.

Further reading

Haverkamp W, Shenasa M, Borggrefe M *et al*. Torsade de pointes. In: Zipes DP, Jalife J, eds. *Cardiac electrophysiology: from cell to bedside*. WB Saunders, 1995: Chapter 79.

Tzivoni D, Banai S, Schuger C *et al*. Treatment of torsade de pointes with magnesium sulfate. *Circulation* 1988;**77**: 392–7.

83 How do I assess the patient with long QT? Should I screen relatives, and how? How do I treat them?

J Benhorin

Patients affected by the congenital long QT syndrome (LQT) are often first assessed when syncope, documented ventricular arrhythmia or aborted cardiac arrest affects them or a family member. The diagnostic cut-offs (<100% sensitive) for a congenitally-prolonged heart rate-corrected QT interval (QTc) on standard 12-lead ECG (measured in lead II, or V5) are: >0.46 sec (children <16 years), >0.45 sec (adult males), and >0.47 sec (adult females), after drug induced QT prolongation has been excluded. T wave morphology should also be carefully examined, in particular for high takeoff, late onset, broad base, bifid morphology with humps, and beat-by-beat alternating polarity (T wave alternans). In several LQT variants, sinus bradycardia is an additional common feature. Holter monitoring should be performed to exclude repetitive ventricular arrhythmias of the torsade de pointes type. Family screening by 12-lead ECG of all first-degree relatives is mandatory in order to have a definite diagnosis of hereditary LQT. In Romano-Ward syndrome (1/20,000 births: autosomal dominant transmission with >90% penetrance), 50% of offspring of one affected parent are predicted to be similarly affected.

Six associated genetic loci (on chromosomes 3, 4, 7, 11, 21, 22) have been identified, of which four relate to genes that encode cardiac ion-channel proteins. Several mutations have been described for each gene. Although only 50% of all LQT affected families can be linked to one of these genes, genetic screening is 100% accurate amongst these, and can provide a definite diagnosis in phenotypically borderline cases.

Medical therapy should be promptly started in symptomatic LQT patients, and beta blockers are currently the first choice, with the occasional need for pacemaker implantation. However, recent evidence suggests that in symptomatic cases with aborted cardiac arrest, automatic implantable cardiac defibrillator (ICD) implantation, in addition to beta blocker therapy, is probably indicated. In patients who do not respond to the above-mentioned measures, high cervicothoracic sympathectomy might be beneficial. Currently, there is no consensus regarding the need for therapy in asymptomatic patients, unless their phenotype is exceedingly abnormal. Gene-specific medical therapy is currently being investigated.

Further Reading

Benhorin J, Taub R, Goldmit M *et al*. Effects of flecainide in patients with a new SCN5A mutation: mutation specific therapy for long QT syndrome? *Circulation* 2000;**101**: 1698–706.

Jiang C, Atkinson D, Towbin JA *et al*. Two long QT syndrome loci map to chromosomes 3 and 7 with evidence for further heterogeneity. *Nat Genet* 1994;**8**: 141–7.

Keating MT, Atkinson D, Dunn C *et al*. Linkage of a cardiac arrhythmia, the long QT syndrome, and the Harvey ras-1 gene. *Science* 1991;**252**: 704–6.

Moss AJ, Schwartz PJ, Crampton RS *et al*. The long QT syndrome: prospective longitudinal study of 328 families. *Circulation* 1991;**84**: 1136–44.

Schott JJ, Charpentier F, Pettier S *et al*. Mapping of a gene for the long QT syndrome to chromosome 4q25–27. *Am J Hum Genet* 1995;**57**: 1114–22.

Schwartz PJ, Priori SG, Locati EH *et al*. Long QT syndrome patients with mutations on the SCN5A and HERG genes have differential responses to Na$^+$ channel blockade and to increases in heart rate: implications for gene-specific therapy. *Circulation* 1995;**92**: 3381–6.

Vincent GM, Timothy KW. The spectrum of symptoms and QT intervals in carriers of the gene for the long QT syndrome. *N Engl J Med* 1992;**327**: 846–52.

84 How do I investigate the relatives of a patient with sudden cardiac death?

Niall G Mahon and W McKenna

In patients aged over 30 years by far the commonest cause of sudden cardiac death is coronary disease (80%). In patients younger than this, inherited disorders play a major role, with hypertrophic cardiomyopathy accounting for approximately 50% of these deaths. Although perhaps not entirely representative of the general population, the most systematically collected data on sudden death in young people comes from athletes. Common causes of sudden death in young athletes are shown in table 84.1. Aortic root dissection and arrhythmias due to accessory pathways and long QT syndromes may also be causative. A specific diagnosis in the deceased should be pursued by means of expert examination of the postmortem heart if available and attempts to obtain ante-mortem electrocardiograms and other investigations.

Table 84.1 Common causes of death in young athletes

Cause of sudden cardiac death in 288 young competitive athletes	% of cases
Hypertrophic cardiomyopathy	51
Anomalous coronary artery	17
Other coronary disease	9
Myocarditis	5
Dilated cardiomyopathy	4
Ruptured aortic aneurysm	3
Aortic valve stenosis	3
Arrhythmogenic right ventricular cardiomyopathy	2
Mitral valve prolapse	2

From Basilico FC. Cardiovascular disease in athletes. *Am J Sports Med* 1999;**27**: 108–21.

In general first-degree relatives should undergo history, physical examination, 12-lead electrocardiography and 2-D echocardiography. Other investigations may also be performed depending on the suspected cause of death, such as exercise testing in suspected long QT syndrome. In the case of a suspected inherited condition, if both parents of the deceased can be evaluated and found to be free of abnormalities, the condition causing death is likely to have been sporadic and the chances of siblings being affected are low. However, this inference must be tempered by the realisation that some inherited conditions (including hypertrophic cardiomyopathy) may be associated with incomplete penetrance. Extended pedigree analyses have demonstrated that occasionally apparently unaffected individuals, termed "obligate carriers", carry the mutation. A follow up strategy after an initial negative evaluation is empirical, and depends on the age of the person, the level of anxiety and the nature of the suspected condition.

Further reading

Basilico FC. Cardiovascular disease in athletes. *Am J Sports Med* 1999;**27**: 108–1.

Corrado D, Basso C, Schiavon M *et al*. Screening for hypertrophic cardiomyopathy in young athletes. *N Engl J Med* 1998;**339**: 364–9.

85 What percentage of patients will suffer the complications of amiodarone therapy, and how reversible are the eye, lung, and liver changes? How do I assess thyroid function in someone on amiodarone therapy?

Daniel E Hillman

Amiodarone therapy is associated with a number of serious toxicities which primarily involve the lung, heart, liver or thyroid gland. The drug is also associated with a wide array of other side effects involving the skin, eye, gastrointestinal tract and neurologic system. Drug discontinuance rates with amiodarone are closely related to its daily dose. The table summarises the cumulative incidence of adverse reactions reported in two separate meta-analyses.[1,2]

Eye, lung, and liver toxicity are all potentially reversible if amiodarone is discontinued early after the development of toxicity. However, cases of permanent blindness, death from liver failure and death from respiratory failure have been rarely reported with amiodarone.

There are no adequate predictors of pulmonary toxicity, and serial lung function studies are usually not helpful. Dose and duration of treatment are no guide to risk. Clinical suspicion must remain high, especially in the elderly or those with co-existent pulmonary disease.[3]

Amiodarone has been implicated as a cause of both hyper-thyroidism and hypothyroidism. Hypothyroidism is a predictable response to the iodide load presented by amiodarone. Two types of hyperthyroidism have been reported to occur with amiodarone. Type I amiodarone-induced hyperthyroidism occurs in patients with underlying thyroid disease such as Graves disease. The iodide load in these patients accelerates thyroid hormone synthesis. Type II amiodarone-induced hyperthyroidism occurs in patients with normal thyroids. Hyperthyroidism results from a direct toxic effect of amiodarone causing a subacute destructive thyroiditis with release of preformed thyroid hormone. Patients receiving amiodarone should have thyroid function evaluated at periodic intervals. A low TSH is indicative of hyperthyroidism, but does not distinguish between Type 1 and Type 2 hyperthyroidism. Radioactive iodine uptake may be low normal or elevated in Type 1 hyperthyroidism but is very low or absent in Type 2 hyperthyroidism. Interleukin-6 levels are normal or moderately increased in Type 1, but markedly increased in Type 2 amiodarone-induced hyperthyroidism. In addition, colour flow Doppler ultrasound shows an absence of vascularity in Type 2 amiodarone-induced hyperthyroidism.

Amiodarone-induced hypothyroidism is characterised by an elevated TSH. Treatment of amiodarone-induced hypothyroidism is indicated if the free T4 is low or low normal and the TSH is greater than 20 microIU/ml.

As a complication of therapy, hyperthyroidism is more common where dietary iodine intake is low, whilst the reverse is true in areas of high intake.[4] In patients with hyperthyroidism in whom amiodarone therapy is still warranted, thought should be given to concomitant treatment with carbimazole.[5]

Table 85.1   Incidence (% and odds ratios) of adverse reactions in two recently published meta-analyses

	ATMI* meta-analysis[1]			Low-dose meta-analysis[2]		
	Amio-darone	Placebo	OR†	Amio-darone	Placebo	OR
Pulmonary	1.6	0.5	3.1	1.9	0.7	2.2
Hepatic	1.0	0.4	2.7	1.2	0.8	1.2
Thyroid	8.4	1.6	4.9	3.7	0.4	4.2
Bradycardia	2.4	0.8	2.6	3.3	1.4	2.2
Neurologic	0.5	0.2	2.8	4.6	1.9	2.0
Skin	NR‡	NR	NR	2.3	0.7	2.5
Eye	NR	NR	NR	1.5	0.1	3.4
Gastrointestinal	NR	NR	NR	4.2	3.3	1.1
Drug Discontinuation	41	27	NR	23	15	NR

*ATMI = Amiodarone Trials Meta-Analysis Investigators; † OR = odds ratio; ‡ NR = not reported

References

1 Amiodarone Trials Meta-Analysis Investigators. Effect of prophylactic amiodarone on mortality after acute myocardial infarction and in congestive heart failure: meta-analysis of individual data from 6500 patients in randomized trials. *Lancet* 1997;**350**: 1417–24.

2 Vorperian VR, Harighurst TC, Miller S *et al*. Adverse effects of low dose amiodarone: a meta-analysis. *J Am Coll Cardiol* 1997;**30**: 791–8.

3 Gleadhill IC, Wise RA, Schonfeld S *et al*. Serial lung function testing in patients treated with amiodarone: a prospective study. *Am J Med* 1989;**86**: 4–10.

4 Martino E, Safran M, Aghini-Lombardi F *et al*. Environmental iodine intake and thyroid dysfunction during chronic amiodarone therapy. *Ann Intern Med* 1984;**101**: 28–34.

5 Davies PH, Franklyn JA, Sheppard MC. Treatment of amiodarone induced thyrotoxicosis with carbimazole alone and continuation of amiodarone. *BMJ* 1992;**305**: 224–5.

86 Who should have a VT stimulation study? What are the risks and benefits?

Roy M John

Contrary to conventional wisdom, a significant number of sudden arrhythmic deaths result from re-entrant ventricular tachycardia that occurs in patients with chronic heart disease in the absence of acute infarction. These arrhythmias can be safely studied in a controlled setting using electrophysiological testing. Programmed electrical stimulation of the ventricle (also termed VT stimulation studies) has a remarkable sensitivity for re-producing monomorphic ventricular tachycardia associated with infarct related myocardial scars and offers a fairly reliable means of identifying patients at risk for sudden death. Patients with LV dysfunction (LV ejection fraction <40%) who are inducible for monomorphic VT have a risk of sudden cardiac death of approximately 30% over the ensuing year.

The patients at highest risk for sudden death include those who have survived a cardiac arrest not occurring in the context of an acute infarction, and those presenting with sustained VT. These patients are best treated with implantable cardiac defibrillators. The role of VT stimulation studies in such patients is primarily to confirm the diagnosis and exclude focal ventricular arrhythmias or unusual supraventricular arrhythmias indistinguishable from VT that are amenable to RF ablation. Occasionally, suppression of VT inducibility with drugs such as amiodarone and sotalol may be an acceptable alternative to implantable cardioverter defibrillator (ICD) implant.

VT stimulation studies are more valuable for patients with severe heart disease and unexplained syncope. Such patients may have had a self-limiting arrhythmia causing their syncope. Inducibility of monomorphic VT is a fairly specific finding in this patient population especially if their heart disease is based on coronary artery disease. In addition, electrophysiological studies can unmask severe His-Purkinje conduction disease requiring pacemaker implantation. One major drawback of VT stimulation studies is the low sensitivity for ventricular arrhythmia in non-ischaemic dilated cardiomyopathy. In these patients, if the clinical suspicion is high, a negative study may well represent a false negative. A second problem with VT studies is the uncertain reliability of induced polymorphic VT or ventricular fibrillation as end points. Recent data from subgroup analysis of the Multicenter Unsustained Tachycardia Trial (MUSTT) suggests that such arrhythmias may be just as important as monomorphic VT for predicting mortality in the face of severe LV dysfunction.

Perhaps the most important role of VT study is in primary prevention of sudden death. Two recent randomised trials have demonstrated conclusively that patients with depressed LV function and non-sustained VT (defined as three or more beats of VT at a rate >120bpm) will benefit from ICD implantation if they are inducible for sustained VT.[1,2] Clinical trials are in progress to determine if ICD implantation would benefit patients with low LVEF and heart failure alone without resorting to an EP study. Pending their results, patients with LV dysfunction who manifest non-sustained VT should undergo VT stimulation studies to see if they would benefit from an ICD. This strategy appears to be cost effective.[3]

The risks of invasive electrophysiological studies are related to venous (and rarely arterial) cannulation and from the arrhythmias induced. Injury to the vascular structures and venous thrombosis occurs rarely (less than 2%). Cardiac perforation from catheter placement is equally rare (0.4%); death from the procedure occurred in 0.12% in one study[4] and underlines the importance of trained personnel and well equipped laboratories for these studies.

References

1 Buxton AE, Lee KL, Fisher JD *et al*. A randomized study of the prevention of sudden death in patients with coronary artery disease. *N Engl J Med* 1999;**341**: 1882–90.
2 Moss AJ, Hall WJ, Cannom DS *et al*. Improved survival with an implanted defibrillator in patients with coronary disease at high risk for ventricular arrhythmia. *N Engl J Med* 1996;**335**: 1933–40.
3 Mushlin AI, Hall WJ, Zwanziger J *et al*. The cost effectiveness of automatic implantable cardiac defibrillators: results from MADIT. Multicenter Automatic Defibrillator Implantation Trial. *Circulation* 1998;**97**: 2129–35.
4 Horowitz L. Safety of electrophysiologic studies. *Circulation* 1986;**73(suppl)**: II28–31.

87 What are the indications for implantable cardioverter defibrillator (ICD) implantation and what are the survival benefits?

Roy M John and Mark Squirrell

Studies in the early 1980s showed that recurrence rates were high for patients presenting with a malignant arrhythmia unrelated to myocardial ischaemia or infarction. Survivors of cardiac arrest, those presenting with sustained monomorphic VT and unexplained syncope in the presence of heart disease clearly are patients at high risk for sudden cardiac death. A series of clinical trials completed in the recent past have confirmed the uniform survival benefit from ICD therapy in such patients (AVID, CASH, CIDS) when compared to therapy with amiodarone or sotalol. In the largest prospective randomised trial (Antiarrhythmics versus Implantable Defibrillators Trial – AVID trial), the ICD reduced mortality by 39% at 1 year and 31% at 3 years. Most patients randomised to the antiarrhythmic arm of the trial were treated with amiodarone.

With remarkable improvements in ICD technology allowing easier implantation, the ICD is being embraced increasingly and earlier in the course of cardiac disease. Attention has now turned to primary prevention of sudden death. For patients with asymptomatic non-sustained VT, there appears to be a clear survival benefit from ICD in the presence of a remote myocardial infarction, LVEF <40%, and inducible VT at electrophysiological study (MADIT, MUSTT). Interestingly, this benefit cannot be extrapolated to patients without non-sustained VT or inducible VT. The CABG patch trial that randomised patients with LVEF <36% and positive signal averaged ECG to ICD or not during elective bypass surgery failed to show a survival benefit. The role of the ICD in primary prevention of sudden death in non-ischaemic dilated cardiomyopathy is also unclear at this time. Clinical trials are in progress.

The benefit from an ICD appears to be greatest for patients with severe LV function and additive to conventional therapy with ACE inhibitors and beta adrenergic blockers. In the AVID trial for example, survival benefit with ICD was observed only when LVEF was less than 35%. Similarly, in the primary prevention trials, the mean LVEF was 30%. One could advance the argument that the ICD should be reserved for those with the worst LV function. Unfortunately, such patients have competing causes for mortality such as pump failure and electromechanical dissociation that are responsible for 50% of deaths. On the other hand, patients with little or no impairment of LV function and a single tachyarrhythmic event usually have late and rare recurrence leading to sudden death. An ICD can potentially restore them to near normal life expectancy in the absence of ongoing myopathic process. The long term studies requiring more than one life span of an ICD are not available to define the true value of ICD therapy in such patients.

Although the ability of the implantable cardioverter defibrillator (ICD) to terminate potentially lethal ventricular arrhythmias is well acknowledged there is less consensus as to whom should receive an ICD. A good place to start is the American College of Cardiology/American Heart Association Practice Guidelines for Arrhythmia Devices.[1] There are three classes of indications: class one, where there is evidence and/or general agreement that the treatment is beneficial, useful and effective; class two, where there is conflicting evidence or a divergence of opinion; and class three, where there is evidence and general agreement that a treatment is not useful or effective.

The class one indications for ICD implantation are:

1 Cardiac arrest due to VF or VT not due to a transient or reversible cause.
2 Spontaneous sustained VT.
3 Syncope of undetermined origin with clinically relevant, haemodynamically significant sustained VT or VF induced at electrophysiological study when drug therapy is ineffective, not tolerated or not preferred.
4 Non-sustained VT with coronary disease, prior MI, LV dysfunction, and inducible VF or sustained VT at electrophysiological study that is not suppressible by a class I antiarrhythmic drug.

The class two indications for ICD implantation are:

1 Cardiac arrest presumed to be due to VF when electrophysiological testing is precluded by other medical conditions.
2 Severe symptoms attributable to sustained ventricular arrhythmias while awaiting cardiac transplantation.

3 Familial or inherited conditions with a high risk for life-threatening ventricular tachyarrhythmia such as long QT syndrome or hypertrophic cardiomyopathy.
4 Non-sustained VT with coronary artery disease, prior MI, and LV dysfunction, and inducible sustained VT or VF at electrophysiological study.
5 Recurrent syncope of undetermined aetiology in the presence of ventricular dysfunction and inducible ventricular arrhythmias at electrophysiological study when other causes of syncope have been excluded.

The size of the risk reduction to patients and the degree of life prolongation are only moderate in the trials showing benefit of ICD over antiarrhythmic therapy. The cost per life year saved is also wildly different in these trials giving us conflicting information, e.g. $22,800 (MADIT) and $114,917 (AVID).

There is a wide variation in implant rates across the world (Table 87.1).

Table 87.1   Number of implants per million/ population in western countries[1]

Country	1996	1997	per million population (1997)
USA	23,407	34,121	120
Germany	1975	3556	45
France	210	420	10
Italy	280	950	16
Netherlands	150	220	9
UK	240	410	7

The UK has one of the lowest implant rates in Western Europe and it is not clear if this is reflective of a conservative approach by UK cardiologists, tight budgetary constraints or a lack of clear clinical trial data. The recently published NICE guidelines, if implemented, will result in an increase in the ICD implantation rate to 50 per million.[2]

In conclusion, a patient who has survived an out of hospital cardiac arrest unrelated to a transient or reversible cause should receive a device irrespective of inducibility at EP study. If this patient has an EF < 35% the case for this is stronger. Patients who have repeated hospital admissions for symptomatic sustained ventricular tachycardia that are not amenable to RF ablation are also clear beneficiaries as well as providing a long term cost saving to the health care system. Other patients must be dealt with on a case by case basis weighing up all the individual circumstances.

Reference
1 Garrett C. A new evidence base for implantable cardioverter defibrillator therapy. *Eur Heart J* 1998;**19**: 189–91.
2 National Institute for Clinical Excellence. *Guidance on the use of implantable cardioverter defibrillators for arrhythmias.* Technology Appraisal Guidance–No. 11, September 2000. (www.nice.org.uk)

Further reading
Bigger JT. Coronary artery bypass grafting (CABG)-patch trial. *N Engl J Med* 1997;**337**: 1569–75.
Gregoratos G, Cheitlin MD, Conill A *et al*. The American College of Cardiology/American Heart Association practice guidelines for arrhythmia devices. *J Am Coll Cardiol* 1998;**31**: 1175–209.
Moss AJ, Hall WJ, Cannom DS *et al*. Improved survival with an implanted defibrillator in patients with coronary disease at high risk for ventricular arrhythmia. The Multi-Center Automated Defibrillator Implantation (MADIT) Trial. *N Engl J Med* 1996;**335**: 1933–40.
Zipes DP *et al*. A comparison of antiarrhythmic-drug therapy with implantable defibrillators in patients resuscitated from near-fatal ventricular arrhythmias. The anti-arrhythmics versus implantable defibrillators (AVID). *N Engl J Med* 1997;**337**: 1576–83.

88 How do I manage the patient with an ICD?

Roy M John

An implantable cardioverter defibrillator (ICD) serves as prophylaxis against sudden collapse and death from rapid ventricular arrhythmias. In general, all ICDs sense the heart rate and provide anti-tachycardia pacing or deliver synchronised (cardioversion) or unsynchronised (defibrillation) shocks. Some of the modern ICDs also incorporate dedicated pacing function; patients with heart block or sinus node disease may be dependent on these devices just like any patient with an implanted cardiac pacemaker.

Like pacemakers, ICDs have to be checked by telemetric interrogation at periodic intervals to confirm integrity of the lead systems and proper function of ICD components including adequacy of battery voltage. Reprogramming of the various parameters that govern pacing, arrhythmia detection and therapy may be necessary from time to time. Such routine follow up, usually undertaken at established arrhythmia centres, should occur at 3 to 6 monthly intervals in the absence of major intercurrent events. Some issues specific to this group of patients can be summarised as follows:

1. Avoid rapid heart rates

In its basic form, arrhythmia detection algorithms of ICDs rely on a programmed heart rate threshold. Once this is exceeded for a defined period of time, the device may deliver therapy irrespective of whether the arrhythmia is of ventricular or supraventricular origin. In a ventricular-based ICD, the shock energy vector is designed primarily to encompass the ventricles. Consequently, atrial arrhythmias may fail to convert such that multiple inappropriate ICD shocks may result. Further, if anti-tachycardia pacing is delivered in the ventricle for an atrial arrhythmia, ventricular arrhythmias may be provoked creating a pro-arrhythmic situation. The newer ICDs incorporate atrial sensing to improve arrhythmia discrimination but it must be remembered that any algorithm that improves specificity for ventricular arrhythmia will entail some loss of sensitivity. Cognisant of the above, it is imperative that atrial arrhythmias are adequately treated in these patients, particularly the paroxysmal form of atrial fibrillation that is commonly associated with rapid rates at its onset. Occasionally, RF ablation of the AV node is necessary. Beta adrenergic blockers should be an integral part of therapy in most ICD patients.

2. Recognise ICD—drug interactions

Antiarrhythmic drugs have the potential for interacting with an ICD in several ways. Drugs such as flecainide and amiodarone can increase pacing and defibrillation thresholds. In patients with a low margin of safety for these parameters, use of these drugs may result in failure of pacing or defibrillation. Secondly, these drugs can slow the rate of ventricular tachycardia below the programmed rate threshold for detection by the ICD; failure of arrhythmia detection can result. Some rarer interactions include alteration of the T wave voltage by drugs or hyperkalaemia resulting in double counting and inappropriate shocks.

3. ICD wound management

As an implanted device, the system is susceptible to infections. Pain and inflammation of the skin over the ICD may herald an infective process. Similarly, unexplained fever, particularly staphylococcal septicaemia may indicate endocarditis involving the leads and/or tricuspid valve.

89 How do I follow up the patient with the implantable cardioverter defibrillator?

Mark Squirrell

Follow up of the patient with an implantable cardioverter de-fibrillator (ICD) demands an integrated team approach. The cardiologist, technical staff and nurses involved should have a wide experience and knowledge of pacemakers and general cardiac electrophysiology. Current generation ICDs do not just shock the heart but provide complex regimens of tachycardia dis-crimination and anti-tachycardia pacing (ATP) as well as single and dual chamber bradycardia therapy.

Routine follow up may occur in a tertiary centre or a local hospital as long as the expert staff and necessary equipment such as programmers and cardiac arrest kit are available. Follow up should start before the device is implanted with an educational programme and support for the patient and immediate family members. Videos, information booklets and meeting other patients with ICDs may be of benefit.

No consensus exists as to the interval between routine follow ups. Previously the patient had to return every month or two to have a capacitor reform. This is not now necessary, as all modern ICDs will undertake this automatically. With most current devices a 3 to 6 month interval is usual but treat each patient according to their individual circumstances.

Good management of the ICD should aim to achieve the following objectives:

1 Monitor the performance of the therapy delivered by the device, look at the success and failure of the programmed regimes and any acceleration of arrhythmias. Use this infor-mation to optimise clinical effectiveness of the programming.
2 Measure necessary parameters of the ICD and leads to ensure correct function. These should include lead impedance, shock coil impedance (if possible non-invasively), battery voltage, charge time, R and P wave amplitudes as well as pacing thresholds.
3 Review the intracardiac electrograms to ensure no inadvertent sensing of noise or other interference.
4 Maximise device longevity by safe and effective reprogramming of parameters.

5 Minimise the risk of complications occurring both from inappropriate therapy delivered to the patient and those associated with wound and pocket infection.[1]

6 Anticipate the elective replacement of the device and plan for this eventuality.

7 Provide a support structure for the patient and their family including advice, counselling and education. Some centres provide a formal patient support group; there are both positive and negative views on this practice.[2,3]

References

1 Troup P, Chapman P, Wetherbee J *et al*. Clinical features of AICD system infections. *Circulation* 1988;**78**:155.

2 Badger JM, Morris PLP. Observations of a support group for automatic implantable cardioverter defibrillator recipients and their spouses. *Heart Lung* 1989;**18**: 238–43.

3 Teplitz L, Egenes KJ, Brask L. Life after sudden death: the development of a support group for automatic implantable cardioverter defibrillator patients. *J Cardiovasc Nurs* 1990;**4**: 20–32.

90 What do I do if an ICD keeps discharging?

Roy M John and Mark Squirrell

Most patients who experience a single ICD shock do so for successful conversion of a malignant ventricular arrhythmia. However, it must be remembered that the default programming in an ICD is designed to maximise sensitivity at the expense of specificity. Consequently, a significant number of ICD shocks can be inappropriate.[1] For example, multiple shocks in quick succession may indicate inappropriate therapy for an atrial arrhythmia or a problem with the rate sensing lead. For this reason, it is important to retrieve the stored data from the device using the appropriate programmer even after a single shock. Evaluation of events stored in the ICD memory shows intracardiac electrograms, far field electrograms and recorded intervals as well as the onset and stability of the tachycardia to determine appropriate or inappropriate therapy. Frequent episodes of ventricular arrhythmia will require antiarrhythmic drugs for suppression; sotalol is often effective as a first line drug in this situation.[2]

The more common reason for multiple ICD shocks is recurrent ventricular arrhythmia. Patients experiencing "storms" of shocks should be adequately sedated, and monitored in a coronary care setting. Intravenous antiarrhythmic drugs should be used for rapid arrhythmia suppression. Electrolyte abnormalities should be sought and promptly corrected. Myocardial ischaemia has to be a serious consideration when recurrent ventricular fibrillation or polymorphic ventricular tachycardia is responsible for shocks. Most episodes of repetitive ventricular tachycardia respond to intravenous drugs such as lidocaine, procainamide or amiodarone allowing for oral loading with an antiarrhythmic agent in a more controlled fashion.

If it becomes apparent that shocks are being delivered inappropriately (e.g. atrial fibrillation with rapid ventricular rates or shocks with no apparent arrhythmia signifying a lead fracture) suppression of ICD function can be achieved by applying a magnet over the ICD generator. Unless specifically programmed to the contrary, one can temporarily disable the sensing circuit of most ICDs during the period that a magnet is held over the ICD generator and prevent unnecessary shock while awaiting availability of appropriate equipment for definitive ICD programming changes.

Other causes of inappropriate therapy include:

- Sinus tachycardia
- Lead fracture
- Diaphragmatic muscle sensing
- Electromagnetic interference.

References
1 Nunain SO, Roelke M, Trouton T *et al*. Limitations and late complications of third-generation automatic cardioverter-defibrillators. *Circulation* 1995;**91**: 2204–13.
2 Pacifico A, Hohnloser SH, Williams JH *et al*. Prevention of implantable-defibrillator shocks by treatment with sotalol. *N Engl J Med* 1999;**340**: 1855–62.

91 How do I manage the pregnant woman with dilated cardiomyopathy?

Sara Thorne

The management of a pregnant woman with dilated cardio-myopathy should be considered in terms of maternal risk, and risk to the fetus.

Maternal risk

This relates to the degree of ventricular dysfunction and the ability to adapt to altered haemodynamics. Risk and management can therefore be discussed in relation to New York Heart Association (NYHA) functional class:

NYHA I-II

- Should manage pregnancy without difficulty (maternal mortality 0.4%)
- May require admission for rest and diuretic therapy
- Venous thrombosis prophylaxis with heparin for patients on bedrest

NYHA III

- At significant risk (maternal mortality for NYHA III-IV 6.8%)
- Planned hospital admission for rest, treatment of heart failure and monitoring
- Risk of deterioration in ventricular function which may not improve post-partum.
- Early delivery if heart failure progressive despite optimal in-patient management

NYHA IV

- Should be advised not to become pregnant. Therapeutic abortion should be considered.

Fetal risk

Fetal risk should be considered in terms of two factors:

1 Factors which put the mother at risk
2 Adverse effects from maternal drugs:
  - ACE inhibitors should be discontinued prior to conception because of the risk of embryopathy
  - Limited or unfavourable data on fetal effects of many antiarryhthmics
  - Beta blockers may be associated with maternal hypotension, and hence reduce placental perfusion. They may thus contribute to premature labour
  - Warfarin – see Q93 (page 196) and Q95 (page 202).

Note that digoxin and verapamil are safe to use.

Further reading
Oakley CM. Management of pre-existing disorders in pregnancy: heart disease. *Presc J* 1997;**37**: 102–11.
Salazar E, Izaguirre R, Verdejo J *et al*. Failure of adjusted doses of subcutaneous doses of heparin to prevent thromboembolic phenomena in pregnant patients with mechanical cardiac valve prostheses. *J Am Coll Cardiol* 1996;**27**: 1698–703.

92 How do I manage the pregnant woman with valve disease?

Sara Thorne

Native or tissue valves

In general, regurgitant lesions are well tolerated during pregnancy, whereas left sided stenotic lesions are not (increased circulating volume and cardiac output lead to a rise in left atrial pressure). Tissue valves can deteriorate rapidly during pregnancy.

Management of patients with significant mitral and aortic stenosis

1 Bedrest:
  - Reduced heart rate allows time for LV filling and ejection
  - Reduced venous return due to IVC compression by the uterus reduces LA pressure (also increases risk of thrombosis: patients must be heparinised).
2 Dyspnoea and angina: slow the heart rate with beta blockers or digoxin. Nitrates may be useful, but should be used with caution in those with aortic stenosis.
3 Intractable pulmonary oedema:
  - Balloon valvotomy
  - Closed mitral valvotomy (advantage as no cardiopulmonary bypass, but few surgeons nowadays have experience)
  - If valvotomy not possible, then deliver fetus by Caesarean section followed by cardiopulmonary bypass and valve replacement.

Mechanical valves

Anticoagulation is the issue here: in particular, the risk of warfarin embryopathy vs risk of valve thrombosis.

The choice lies between:

1 Warfarin throughout pregnancy, stopping it for a minimal length of time for delivery
2 Convert to heparin during the first trimester with hospital admission and meticulous control of APTT. Return to warfarin for the second trimester and reinstate heparin at ~34/40.

Note:

1 Mitral tilting disc prostheses at particular risk: fatal thrombotic occlusion of these valves in pregnant women described despite well-controlled heparin anticoagulation
2 Risk of significant warfarin embryopathy not as high as previously thought, especially if the mother achieves adequate anticoagulation on <5mg warfarin.
3 No data on low molecular weight heparin in this situation, so its use cannot be recommended.

The patient must be fully informed, and involved in deciding her mode of anticoagulation (medicolegal implications).

Further reading

Salazar E, Izaguirre R, Verdejo J *et al.* Failure of adjusted doses of sub-cutaneous doses of heparin to prevent thromboembolic phenomena in pregnant patients with mechanical cardiac valve prostheses. *J Am Coll Cardiol* 1996;**27**: 1698–703.

93 Which cardiac patients should never get pregnant? Which cardiac patients should undergo elective Caesarean section?

Sara Thorne

Which women should never get pregnant?

1 Those with significant pulmonary hypertension (pulmonary vascular resistance >2/3 of systemic), especially cyanotic patients and those with Eisenmenger reaction (maternal mortality ~50%) and those with residual pulmonary hypertension after e.g. VSD closure. NB: Even women with modest pulmonary vascular disease ~1/2 systemic are at risk of death.

2 Those with grade 4 systemic ventricular function (EF <20%).

Which women should not get pregnant until operated upon?

1 Marfan's syndrome patients with aortic aneurysm/dilated aortic root.

2 Those with severe left sided obstructive lesions (AS, MS, coarctation).

Which women should undergo elective Caesarean section?

1 Those with independent obstetric indications.

2 Caesarean section should be strongly considered for the following women:

- Those with mechanical valves, especially tilting disc in the mitral position. The key here is to leave the mother off warfarin for the minimum time possible. An elective section is performed at 38 weeks' gestation, replacing the warfarin with unfractionated heparin for the minimum time possible

- Severe aortic or mitral stenosis.

If the mother's life is at risk, section followed by valve replacement may be necessary.

Controversy remains over whether the following patients should undergo elective Caesarean section:

1 Cyanotic congenital heart disease with impaired fetal growth. Section may help to avoid further fetal hypoxaemia, but at the

expense of excessive maternal haemorrhage to which cyanotic patients are prone.

2 Pulmonary hypertension. See comments above.

A balance has to be made between a spontaneous vaginal delivery with the mother in the lateral decubitus position to attenuate haemodynamic fluctuations, forceps assistance and the smaller volume of blood lost during this type of delivery, and the controlled timing of an elective section. **Probably more important than the route of delivery is peri-partum planning and teamwork:** delivery must be planned in advance, and the patient intensively monitored, kept well hydrated and not allowed to drop her systemic vascular resistance. Consultant obstetric and anaesthetic staff experienced in these conditions should be present, and the cardiologist readily available.

Further reading

Connelly MS, Webb GD, Someville J *et al*. Canadian consensus conference on adult congenital heart disease. *Can J Cardiol* 1998;**14**: 395–452.
Oakley CM. Management of pre-existing disorders in pregnancy: heart disease. *Presc J* 1997;**37**: 102–11.

94 A patient is on life-long warfarin and wishes to become pregnant. How should she be managed?

Rachael James

All anticoagulant options during pregnancy are associated with potential risks to the mother and fetus. Any woman on warfarin who wishes to become pregnant should ideally be seen for pre-pregnancy counselling and should be involved in the anti-coagulation decision as much as possible. Potential risks to the fetus need to be balanced against the increased maternal thrombotic risk during pregnancy. Anticoagulation for mechanical heart valves in pregnancy remains an area of some controversy.

The use of warfarin during pregnancy is associated with a low risk of maternal complications[1] but it readily crosses the placenta and embryopathy can follow exposure between 6–12 weeks' gestation, the true incidence of which is unknown. A single study has reported that a maternal warfarin dose ≤5mg is without this embryopathy risk.[2] As pregnancy progresses, the immature vitamin K metabolism of the fetus can result in intracranial haemorrhage even when the maternal INR is well controlled. In addition, a direct CNS effect of warfarin has been described, resulting in structural abnormalities. Conversion to heparin in the final few weeks of pregnancy is recommended to prevent the delivery of, what is in effect, an anticoagulated fetus.[3]

In contrast, unfractionated heparin (UFH) is free from direct fetal harm but it has varied pharmacokinetic and anticoagulant effects and adequate maternal anticoagulation can be difficult to achieve. The use of UFH in women with mechanical valve replacements during pregnancy has been associated with increased maternal thrombosis and bleeding. Studies have been criticised for the use of inadequate heparin dosing and/or inadequate therapeutic ranges[4] although a recent prospective study which used heparin in the first trimester and in the final weeks of pregnancy reported fatal valve thromboses despite adequate anticoagulation.[5] Long term heparin use risks osteoporosis and heparin-induced thrombocytopenia (HIT).[4] Intensive monitoring is required in pregnancy and the use of anti-Xa assays may be necessary.

Low molecular weight heparins (LMWH) have a more reliable anticoagulant effect.[6] The dose is adjusted according to anti-Xa levels. Use in pregnancy is mainly for thromboprophylaxis rather than full anticoagulation but experience is increasing. Indeed, case reports are starting to emerge where LMWH has been used for mechanical valve replacements. Compared with UFH the risk of HIT and osteoporosis are reduced[6] and these heparins may hold the future for anticoagulation in pregnancy.

Management

Women who do not wish to continue warfarin throughout pregnancy can be reassured that conceiving on warfarin appears safe but conversion to heparin, to avoid the risk of embryopathy, needs to be carried out by 6 weeks. Breast-feeding on either warfarin or heparin is safe. Possible regimes include:

- Warfarin throughout pregnancy until near term and then conversion to unfractionated heparin.
- Unfractionated heparin for the first trimester. Warfarin until near term and then resumption of heparin.

References
1 Oakley CM. Anticoagulants in pregnancy. *Br Heart J* 1995;**74**: 107–11.
2 Cotrufo M, de Luca TSL, Calabro R *et al*. Coumarin anticoagulation during pregnancy in patients with mechanical valve prostheses. *Eur J Cardiothorac Surg* 1991;**5**: 300–5.
3 Maternal and Neonatal Haemostasis Working Party of the Haemostasis and Thrombosis Task Force. Guidelines on the prevention, investigation and management of thrombosis associated with pregnancy. *J Clin Pathol* 1993;**46**: 489–96.
4 Ginsberg JS, Hirsh J. Use of antithrombotic agents during pregnancy. *Chest* 1995;**108(suppl 4)**: 305S–11S.
5 Salazar E, Izaguirre R, Verdejo J *et al*. Failure of adjusted doses of subcutaneous heparin to prevent thromboembolic phenomena in pregnant patients with mechanical cardiac valve prostheses. *J Am Coll Cardiol* 1996;**27**: 1698–703.
6 Hirsh J. Low-molecular weight heparin for the treatment of venous thromboembolism. *Am Heart J* 1998;**135(suppl 6)**: S336–42.

95 How should the anticoagulation of a patient with a mechanical heart valve be managed for elective surgery?

Matthew Streetly

Mechanical heart valves are associated with an annual risk of arterial thromboembolism of <8%. Although warfarin greatly reduces the risk, it is at the expense of an INR-related risk of serious haemorrhage. This constitutes an unacceptable risk for patients undergoing major surgery, and it is necessary to temporarily institute alternative anticoagulant measures.

The anticoagulant effect of oral warfarin is prolonged (half life 36 hours) and it can take 3–5 days for a therapeutic INR to fall to less than 1.5. It is also dependent on the half life of the vitamin K dependent clotting factors (particularly factors X and II, with half lives of 36 and 72 hours respectively). The surgical procedure must therefore be planned with this in mind. A "safe" INR depends on the surgery being undertaken. An INR <1.5 is usually suitable, although this should be <1.2 for neurosurgical and ophthalmic procedures.

Four days prior to surgery warfarin should be stopped. Once the INR falls below a therapeutic level heparin should be started. Unfractionated heparin (UFH) should be administered as an intravenous infusion. It has a short lasting effect (half life 2 to 4 hours) and is monitored using daily measurements of the APTT ratio (aim for APTT 1.5–2.5 times greater than control APTT). Alternatively, a weight-adjusted dose of low molecular weight heparin (LMWH) is given subcutaneously once daily with predictable anticoagulant effect, although data are limited. The night prior to surgery the INR should be checked and if it is inappropriately high then surgery should be delayed. If surgery cannot be delayed, the effect of warfarin can be reversed by fresh frozen plasma (2–4 units) or a small dose of intravenous vitamin K (0.5–2mg). Six hours prior to surgery heparin should be stopped to allow the APTT to fall to normal.

Recommencing intravenous heparin in the immediate postoperative period may increase the risk of haemorrhage to greater levels than the risk of thromboembolism with no anticoagulation. Heparin is usually restarted 12–24 hours after surgery, depending on the type of surgery and the cardiac reason for warfarin. Each case must be considered individually. Warfarin should be restarted as soon as the patient is able to tolerate oral medication. Prophylactic heparin should be stopped once an INR greater than 2.0 is established.

Further reading
Ansell J. Oral anticoagulants for the treatment of venous thrombolism. *Ball Clin Haematol* 1998;**11**: 647–50.
Haemostasis and Thrombosis Task Force. Guidelines on oral anticoagulation: third edition. *Br J Haematol* 1998;**101**: 374–87.
Kearon C. Perioperative management of long-term anticoagulation. *Semin Thromb Haem* 1998;**24 (suppl 1)**: 77–83.
Kearon C, Hirsch J. Management of anticoagulation before and after elective surgery. *N Engl J Med* 1997;**336**: 1506–11.

96 What are the indications for surgical management of endocarditis?

Marc R Moon

The indications for surgical management of endocarditis fall into six categories.

1. Congestive heart failure

Patients with moderate-to-severe heart failure require urgent surgical intervention. With mitral regurgitation, afterload reduction and diuretic therapy can improve symptoms and may make it possible to postpone surgical repair until a full course of antibiotic therapy has been completed. In contrast, acute aortic regurgitation progresses rapidly despite an initial favourable response to medical therapy, and early surgical intervention is imperative.

2. Persistent sepsis

This is defined as failure to achieve bloodstream sterility after 3–5 days of appropriate antibiotic therapy or a lack of clinical improvement after one week.

3. Recognised virulence of the infecting organism

- With *native valve* endocarditis, streptococcal infections can be cured with medical therapy in 90%. However, *S. aureus* and gram negative bacteria are more aggressive, requiring trans-oesophageal echocardiography to rule out deep tissue invasion or subtle valvular dysfunction. Fungal infections invariably require surgical intervention
- With *prosthetic valve* endocarditis, streptococcal tissue valve infections involving *only* the leaflets can be cleared in 80% with antibiotic therapy alone; however, mechanical or tissue valve infections involving the sewing ring generally require valve replacement. If echocardiography demonstrates a perivalvular leak, annular extension, or a large vegetation, early operation is necessary

4. Extravalvular extension

Annular abscesses are more common with aortic (25-50%) than mitral (1-5%) infections; in either case, surgical intervention is preferred (survival: 25% medical, 60-80% surgical). Conduction disturbances are a typical manifestation.

5. Peripheral embolisation

This is common (30-40%), but the incidence falls dramatically following initiation of antibiotic therapy. Medical therapy is appropriate for asymptomatic aortic or small vegetations. Surgical therapy is indicated for recurrent or multiple embolisation, large mobile mitral vegetations or vegetations that increase in size despite appropriate medical therapy.

6. Cerebral embolisation

Operation within 24 hours of an infarct carries a 50% exacerbation and 67% mortality rate, but the risk falls after two weeks (exacerbation <10%, mortality <20%). Following a bland infarct, it is ideal to wait 2–3 weeks unless haemodynamic compromise obligates early surgical intervention. Following a haemorrhagic infarct, operation should be postponed as long as possible (4–6 weeks).

Further reading
Moon MR, Stinson EB, Miller DC. Surgical treatment of endocarditis. *Prog Cardiovasc Dis* 1997;**40**: 239–64.

97 What is the morbidity and mortality of endocarditis with modern day management (and how many relapse)?

Peter Wilson

Despite progress in management, morbidity and mortality remain major problems for the patient with endocarditis, both during the acute phase and as the result of long term complications after a bacteriological cure. Improvements in microbiological diagnosis, types of antibiotic treatment and timing of surgical intervention have improved the outlook for some patients but the impact has been minor with some of the more invasive pathogens. The infection can relapse and vegetations can be reinfected. Healed vegetations may leave valvular function so compromised that surgery is required.

In 140 patients with acute infective endocarditis, 48 (34%) required valve replacement during treatment.[1] Heart failure occurred in 46 patients. During the active disease, 22 patients (16%) died. Medical treatment alone cured 80 patients. Relapse occurred in 3 (2.7%) of 112 patients all within one month of discharge. Recurrence was observed in 5 (4%) patients between 4 months and 15 years after the first episode. In the follow up period, another 16 patients died of cardiac causes, most within five years. Of 34 patients with late prosthetic valve endocarditis, 27 (79%) survived their hospital admission but 11 had further surgery during the next five years, usually following cardiac failure.[2] In another study, 91 (70%) of 130 patients survived hospitalisation for native valve endocarditis and 17 of 60 initially treated medically required surgery during a mean 9 year follow up.[3] During follow up, 29 (22%) patients died, 13 from cardiac causes.

References

1 Tornos P, Sanz E, Permanyer-Miralda G *et al*. Late prosthetic valve endocarditis. Immediate and long term prognosis. *Chest* 1992;**101**: 37–41.

2 Tornos MP, Permanyer-Miralda G, Olona M *et al*. Long-term complications of native valve infective endocarditis in non-addicts. *Ann Intern Med* 1992;**117**: 567–72.

3 Verheul HA, Van Den Brink RBA, Van Vreeland T *et al*. Effects of changes in management of active infective endocarditis on outcome in a 25 year period. *Am J Cardiol* 1993;**72**: 682–7.

98 What percentage of blood cultures will be positive in endocarditis?

Peter Wilson

The great majority of patients with endocarditis have positive blood cultures within a few days of incubation and only a few cases will become positive on further incubation for 1–2 weeks. The proportion of culture-negative cases depends on the volume of blood and method of culture but a common estimate is 5% with a range from 2.5% to 31%.[1] Most cases of culture-negative endocarditis are related to use of antibiotics within the preceding two weeks and probably represent infections with staphylococci, streptococci or enterococci. If antibiotics have been given, withdrawal of treatment for four days and serial blood cultures will usually demonstrate the pathogen.

A number of organisms may grow only if incubated under the correct conditions. Nutritionally-deficient streptococci may fail to grow in ordinary media and yet are part of the normal mouth flora and can cause endocarditis.[2] The HACEK organisms are slow growing and easily missed. *Coxiella burnetti, Chlamydia spp.* and *Mycoplasma spp.* are rare causes of endocarditis and are difficult to grow, diagnosis requiring biopsy or serology. *Bartonella spp.* are now known to cause endocarditis in homeless patients and diagnosis is difficult by conventional methods.[3]

Three sets of blood cultures will demonstrate at least 95% of culturable organisms causing endocarditis. After four negative cultures there is only a 1% chance of an organism being identified by later culture.[4] Contamination as the result of poor collection technique makes interpretation difficult and is a greater risk when repeated sets of culture are collected.

References

1 Barnes PD, Crook DWM. Culture negative endocarditis. *J Infect* 1997;**35**: 209–13.

2 Stein DS, Nelson KE. Endocarditis due to nutritionally deficient streptococci: therapeutic dilemma. *Rev Infect Dis* 1987;**9**: 908–16.

3 Raoult D, Fournier PE, Drancourt M *et al*. Diagnosis of 22 new cases of Bartonella endocarditis. *Ann Intern Med* 1996;**125**: 646–52

4 Aronson MD, Bor DH. Blood cultures. *Ann Intern Med* 1987;**106**: 246–53.

99 Which patients should receive antibiotic prophylaxis for endocarditis, and which procedures should be covered in this way?

Peter Wilson

There is little firm scientific evidence for present advice on antibiotic prophylaxis for endocarditis, mainly because of the rarity of the disease. Only 10% of cases are related to bacteraemia caused by invasive procedures. Prevention of endocarditis in patients with abnormal heart valves can be achieved by many general measures, for example, regular dental care. The convention for the use of antibiotics in the prevention of endocarditis derives from animal models and clinical experience. Although dental extraction results in a bacteraemia of about 100cfu/mL, no obvious relationship has been found between the number of circulating bacteria and the likelihood of developing endocarditis.

In man, case-control studies suggest 17% of cases might be prevented if prophylaxis is given for all procedures in patients with abnormal valves.[1] Individual cases of endocarditis following dental or urological procedures have been reported but the risk of developing endocarditis must be very low. Underlying cardiac abnormalities greatly increase the risk of endocarditis, e.g. patent ductus arteriosus, prosthetic valves, hypertrophic cardiomyopathy, aortic valve disease or previous endocarditis. Mitral valve prolapse is common but merits antibiotic prophylaxis if it causes a murmur.

Procedures causing gingival bleeding should be covered by prophylaxis as should tonsillectomy, adenoidectomy and dental work. Other procedures in which prophylaxis should be used include oesophageal dilatation or surgery or endoscopic laser procedures, sclerosis of oesophageal varices, abdominal surgery, instrumentation of ureter or kidney, surgery of prostate or urinary tract. Flexible bronchoscopy with biopsy, cardiac catheterisation, endoscopy with biopsy, liver biopsy, endotracheal intubation and urethral catheterisation in the absence of infection do not need prophylaxis. Patients having colonoscopy or sigmoidoscopy probably do not require prophylaxis unless there is a prosthetic valve or previous endocarditis or unless biopsy is likely to be performed. Recommendations for prophylaxis in patients undergoing obstetric or gynaecological procedures are required for patients with prosthetic valves, or who have previously had endocarditis.

Recommendations for prophylaxis vary between countries. Dental (causing gingival bleeding), oropharyngeal, gastro-intestinal and urological procedures are usually considered a risk.[2] The use of antibiotic prophylaxis is routine during cardiac surgery, flucloxacillin, plus an aminoglycoside, or a cephalosporin being common choices.

References

1 Van Der Meer JTM, Van Wijk W, Thompson J *et al*. Efficacy of antibiotic prophylaxis for prevention of native valve endocarditis. *Lancet* 1992;**339**: 135–9.
2 Leport C, Horstkotte D, Burckhardt D, and the group of experts of the International Society for Chemotherapy. Antibiotic prophylaxis for infective endocarditis from an international group of experts towards a European consensus. *Eur Heart J* 1995;**16(suppl B)**: 126–31.

Further reading

Dajani AS, Bisno AL, Chung KJ *et al*. Prevention of bacterial endo-carditis. Recommendations by the American Heart Association. *JAMA* 1990;**264**: 2919–22.

100 Which patients should undergo preoperative non-invasive investigations or coronary angiography?

Matthew Barnard

Non-invasive testing refers to investigations other than angiography such as dipyridamole thallium scanning or dobutamine stress echocardiography. The literature on this question is overwhelming. It is best approached by nine simple steps. These are based on the recommendations of the joint consensus conference of the American College of Cardiology and the American Heart Association.[1] Clinical predictors, functional capacity and magnitude of surgical risk can be assessed from Tables 101.3, 101.4 and 101.5 in the next question.

Step 1 What is the urgency of surgery?

If absolute emergency proceed to surgery, otherwise proceed to step 2.

Step 2 Has the patient undergone coronary revascularisation in the last five years?

If so and symptoms are stable, proceed to surgery. If not, or symptoms are unstable go to step 3.

Step 3 Has there been a coronary evaluation in the past two years?

If so and there are no changes or new symptoms proceed to surgery. If not, or there have been changes go to step 4.

Step 4 Is there an unstable coronary syndrome or major clinical predictor of risk?

If so proceed direct to angiography. If not go to step 5.

Step 5 Are there intermediate clinical predictors of risk?

If so go to step 6. If not go to step 7.

Step 6 What is the functional capacity and magnitude of surgical risk?

If there are intermediate clinical predictors, then order non-invasive investigations if there is either poor function or high surgical risk. Otherwise go to surgery.

Step 7 Are there minor clinical predictors?

If so go to step 8. If not proceed to surgery.

Step 8 What is the functional capacity and magnitude of surgical risk?

If there are minor clinical predictors, then order non-invasive investigations if there are both poor function and high surgical risk.

Step 9

All patients have now been assigned to surgery, angiography or non-invasive testing. The results of non-invasive tests must incorporate both the absolute result (positive or negative) and quantification of the result (e.g. magnitude and regional location of ischaemic area). These results will determine which patients should proceed to angiography. Significant abnormalities require further assessment by angiography. Minor and intermediate abnormalities only require further assessment in the presence of low functional capacity or major surgical risk.

It should be noted that, at least in high-risk patients undergoing vascular surgery, beta blockade is the only medical intervention proven to have major impact on outcome.[2]

Reference

1 ACC/AHA guidelines for perioperative cardiovascular evaluation for noncardiac surgery. *Circulation* 1996;**93**: 1280–1317.
2 Poldermans D, Boersma E, Bax JJ *et al*. The effect of bisoprolol on perioperative mortality and myocardial infarction in high-risk patients undergoing vascular surgery. Dutch Echocardiographic Cardiac Risk. *N Engl J Med* 1999;**341**: 1789–94.

101 Which factors predict cardiac risk from general surgery and what is the magnitude of the risks associated with each factor?

Matthew Barnard

Mangano and colleagues reported an in-hospital adverse cardiac event rate of 17.5% among patients undergoing major non-cardiac surgery.[1] Four factors require consideration:

1 Clinical predictors
2 Functional status
3 Surgical magnitude
4 Results of non-invasive investigations.

  Clinical risk factors have been integrated into clinical risk scores, of which the best known are the Goldman, Detsky and Eagle scores (Table 101.1).[2] Detsky and colleagues have reported the likelihood of post-testing adverse cardiac events for these scores (Table 101.2).[3] The American Heart Association has classified clinical risk factors into three categories (Table 101.3), based on the conclusions of a consensus conference.[4] This index retains the greatest clinical utility.

  Functional capacity determines the need for non-invasive testing in the presence of intermediate or minor clinical predictors. Daily activities can be scored according to estimated energy expenditure (Table 101.4). The magnitude of the surgical procedure also influences risk (Table 101.5). High surgical risk combined with intermediate clinical risk factors or minor clinical risk factors plus low functional capacity dictate the need for non-invasive testing.

  It is vital to understand that the positive and negative predictive value of non-invasive tests (e.g. thallium scans and dobutamine stress echocardiography) depend critically on the underlying prevalence of cardiac disease in the population. Very low or very high levels of ischaemic heart disease diminish the value of these tests, which are most useful in groups with intermediate levels of disease.[5]

Table 101.1   Clinical risk scoring systems*

	Goldman	Points	Detsky	Points	Eagle**	Points
Age	>70	5	>70	5	>70	1
MI or Q wave	<6 months	10	< 6 months	10	Q wave	1
Angina			CCS class 3	10	Angina	1
			CCS class 4	20		
LV	S3 or raised	11	Pulmonary	10		
dysfunction	JVP		oedema			
			<1 week			
Arrhythmia	Non sinus	7	Non sinus	5	Ventricular	1
					ectopy	
Other heart	Important	3	Critical aortic	20		
disease	Aortic Stenosis		Stenosis			
Other	PO2<60	3	PO2<60	5	Diabetes	1
	pCO2>50		PCO2>50			
	K<3		K<3			
	Urea >50		Urea >50			
	Creatinine >200		Creatinine >260			
			Bedridden			
Surgery	Emergency,	4	Emergency	10		
	Intrathoracic,	3				
	Abdominal					

*Modified from Mangano DT, Golman L. Preoperative assessment of patients with known or suspected coronary artery disease. *N Engl J Med* 1995;**333**: 1750–6.
**Designed for patients undergoing vascular surgery

Table 101.2   Probability of cardiac event by risk score*

Class	Points	Probability of cardiac event (%)
Goldman		
Class 1	0–5	1–8
Class 2	6–12	3–30
Class 3	13–25	14–38
Class 4	>25	30–100
Detsky		
Class 1	0–15	5
Class 2	20–30	27
Class 3	>30	60
Eagle		
Class 1	0	0–3
Class 2	1–2	6–16
Class 3	>3	29–50

*Modified from Palda VA, Detsky AS. Perioperative assessment and management of risk from coronary artery disease. *Ann Intern Med* 1997;**127**: 313–28.

Table 101.3   Clinical predictors of increased cardiovascular risk*

Major
- Unstable coronary syndromes
- Recent MI
- Unstable angina
- Decompensated heart failure
- Significant arrhythmias
- High grade atrioventricular block
- Symptomatic ventricular arrhythmias or supraventricular arryhthmias in presence of underlying heart disease or with uncontrolled ventricular rate
- Severe valvular disease

Intermediate
- Mild stable angina
- Prior MI
- Compensated or previous heart failure
- Diabetes

Minor
- Advanced age
- Abnormal ECG
- Rhythm other than sinus
- Low functional capacity
- History of stroke
- Uncontrolled systemic hypertension

*Modified from ACC/AHA guidelines for perioperative cardiovascular evaluation for noncardiac surgery. *Circulation* 1996;**93**: 1280–317.

Table 101.4   Estimated energy expenditure*

1 MET = resting oxygen consumption of 40 year old 70kg male

1 MET
Eat, dress, use toilet
Walk 50 to 100 metres
Light housework

4 MET
Climb one flight stairs
Run short distance
Heavy housework

10 MET
Strenuous sports

*Modified from ACC/AHA guidelines for perioperative cardiovascular evaluation for noncardiac surgery. *Circulation* 1996;**93**: 1280–317.

Table 101.5   Risk by magnitude of surgery*

High
- Emergent major operations
- Aortic and other vascular surgery
- Anticipated prolonged surgery associated with large fluid shifts

Intermediate
- Carotid endarterectomy
- Head and neck
- Intraperitoneal and intrathoracic
- Orthopaedic
- Prostate

Low
- Endoscopic procedures
- Superficial procedures
- Breast

*Modified from ACC/AHA guidelines for perioperative cardiovascular evaluation for noncardiac surgery. *Circulation* 1996;**93**: 1280–317.

References

1 Mangano DT, Browner WS, Hollenberg M *et al*. Association of perioperative myocardial ischemia with cardiac morbidity and mortality in men undergoing noncardiac surgery. The Study of Perioperative Ischemia Research Group. *N Engl J Med* 1990;**323**: 1781–8.
2 Mangano DT, Golman L. Preoperative assessment of patients with known or suspected coronary artery disease. *N Engl J Med* 1995;**333**: 1750–6.
3 Palda VA, Detsky AS. Perioperative assessment and management of risk from coronary artery disease. *Ann Intern Med* 1997;**127**: 313–28.
4 ACC/AHA guidelines for perioperative cardiovascular evaluation for noncardiac surgery. *Circulation* 1996;**93**: 1280–317.
5 L'Italien GJ, Paul DS, Hendel RC *et al*. Development and validation of a Bayesian model for perioperative cardiac risk assessment in a cohort of 1081 vascular surgical candidates. *J Am Coll Cardiol* 1996;**27**: 779–86.

Index

Main topics of questions are indicated by page references in bold